Springer Series on Geriatric Nursing

Mathy D. Mezey, EdD, RN, FAAN, Series Editor
New York University Division of Nursing

Advisory Board: Margaret Dimond, PhD RN, FAAN; Steven H. Ferris, PhD; Terry Fulmer, PhD RN, FAAN; Linda Kaeser, PhD RN, ACSW, FAAN; Virginia Kayser-Jones, PhD RN, FAAN; Eugenia Siegler, MD; Neville E. Strumpf, PhD RN, FAAN; May Wykle, PhD RN, FAAN; Mary K. Walker, PhD, RN, FAAN

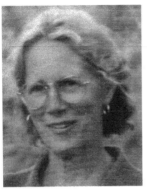

Ann Schmidt Luggen, PhD, RN, MSN, CS, BC-ARNP, CNAA, is Professor of Nursing at Northern Kentucky University. She has a doctoral degree in gerontology and oncology nursing, and a master's degree in oncology nursing, both from the University of Cincinnati. She has also completed a post-master's Geriatric Nurse Practitioner Program at Northern Kentucky University. Dr. Luggen is past President of the National Gerontological Nursing Association, and past Editor of its national newsletter. She is currently President of the Ohio Geriatric Nurse Practitioner Association, and serves on several boards, such as Cincinnati's Nurse Executives, and on the Greater Cincinnati Gerontological Nursing Association. She has written numerous journal articles and books, including *NGNA Core Curriculum for Gerontological Nursing,* which won an AJN Book-of-the-Year award. She lives on a farm in Cincinnati, Ohio with her son and husband, who is a rheumatologist.

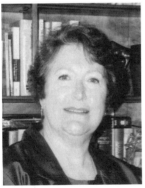

Sue E. Meiner, EdD, APRN, BC, GNP, is an Assistant Professor of Nursing at the University of Nevada-Las Vegas, and a Gerontological Nurse Practitioner at the Clark County Health District in Las Vegas. She received her BSN and MSN degrees at St. Louis University (Missouri), her EdD at Southern Illinois University at Edwardsville, and certification as a Gerontological Nurse Practitioner at Jewish Hospital College of Nursing in St. Louis, Missouri. Prior to her current positions she was Project Director for an NIH and NIA grant at Washington University in St. Louis, School of Medicine, and Associate Professor at the Jewish Hospital College of Nursing and Allied Health. Dr. Meiner authored the book, *Nursing Documentation: Legal Focus Across Practice Settings.* She is co-author with Ann Luggen of three previous books, NGNA Core Curricula for both gerontological nurses and gerontological advanced practice nurses, and *Handbook for the Care of the Older Adult With Cancer.* She is also the author of numerous book chapters and journal articles. Dr. Meiner held an elected political office in St. Louis County for five years in the 1980s and remains active in community service.

Care of
Arthritis
in the
Older Adult

Ann Schmidt Luggen
Sue E. Meiner
Editors

 Springer Publishing Company

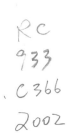
Springer Publishing Company, Inc.
536 Broadway
New York, NY 10012-3955

Acquisitions Editor: Ruth Chasek
Production Editor: Jeanne Libby
Cover design by Joanne E. Honigman

01 02 03 04 05 / 5 4 3 2 1

Library of Congress Cataloging-in-Publication-Data

Care of arthritis in the older adult / Ann Schmidt Luggen,
   Sue E. Meiner, editors.
       p. cm.—(Springer series on geriatric nursing)
     Includes bibliographical references and index.
     ISBN 0-8261-2362-7
     1. Arthritis-Nursing. 2. Geriatric nursing. I. Luggen, Ann
Schmidt. II. Meiner, Sue. III. Series.

RC933 C366 2002
618.97'6722—dc21

                                      2002020929

Printed in Canada by Tri-Graphic.

I dedicate this book to my husband, Michael, who is a rheumatologist, and who has helped me understand the depth and complexity of these many diseases, the arthridites. Further, he has helped me over the years with most of my books, reviewing and critiquing, and was most helpful in reviewing this book.

—Ann Schmidt Luggen

As I was growing up, I watched my grandmother and mother deal with arthritis. Since becoming a nurse nearly 40 years ago, I have cared for thousands of adults with arthritis. Now in my late fifties, I have arthritis. Writing and editing this book was an important component of my personal growth through exploring all avenues of information related to the many facets of this disease. I dedicate this book to all of those people who have been touched by arthritis personally or through family, friends, patients, or acquaintances. I hope a cure for musculoskeletal disorders will occur in the coming decades. In the meantime, this book will provide salient information to those seeking knowledge of caring for the older adult with arthritis.

—Sue E. Meiner

Contents

Contributors

Phyllis J. Atkinson, MS, RN, CS, GNP
St. Elizabeth Medical Center
Family Practice Center
Edgewood, Kentucky

Patricia Birchfield, DSN, ARNP, CS, GNP
Professor
Eastern Kentucky University
Lexington, Kentucky

Catherine A. Hill, MSN, RN, CS, ONC, CEN
Medicine Associates of North Texas
School of Nursing
University of Texas at Arlington
Arlington, Texas

Laurie Kennedy-Malone, PhD, RN, CS
Associate Professor, School of Nursing
University of North Carolina at Greensboro
Greensboro, North Carolina

Patricia Mezinskis, MSN, RN, CS
Associate Professor
University of Cincinnati
Raymond Walters College
Cincinnati, Ohio

Ann Mabe Newman, DSN, RN, CS
Associate Professor of Nursing
Adjunct Associate Professor of Women's Studies
University of North Carolina at Charlotte
Charlotte, North Carolina

Mary R. Painter-Romanello, MSN, RN, GNP
Adult/Geriatric Nurse Practitioner
Good Samaritan Hospital
Cincinnati, Ohio

Barbara Resnick, PhD, CRNP, FAAN, FAANP
Associate Professor
University of Maryland School of Nursing
Baltimore, Maryland

Foreword

Arthritic conditions have often been placed under one huge umbrella which induces us to believe that all are similar, universal and a normal part of aging like skin wrinkles. This text erodes these myths. The arthritic disorders are numerous and symptoms are often no respecter of age and may inexplicably occur. Arthritic disorders cut across all cultures, settings, and ages. Many involve acute exacerbations as well as long remissions. They tend to be ignored by professionals because of our impotence in predicting or assuaging these lingering, chronically debilitating disorders. Every nurse will need this text and particularly those who deal with elders.

Because of the variations of these disorders and marked fluctuations in symptomatology, patients are vulnerable to hoaxes and innocuous therapies. This text deals very prudently with alternative therapies as management strategies.

Quality of life issues are fundamental to any comprehensive nursing care plan and these are dealt with thoughtfully. The commonalities of these disorders are dwarfed by the particulars, but all involve pain and pain management. The authors have dealt with this fundamental issue in depth as one of the most important aspects of arthritis management.

Drs. Luggen and Meiner have special qualifications for producing this text. They have long been involved with a network of rheumatologists and nurse practitioner specialists in the management of rheumatic disorders, and have personal experience with arthritis within their families. Their book includes a holistic perspective, practical management methods, and the contributions of highly qualified nurses. The editors' competence and compassion shine through as we examine this text. It is a pleasure to see this vital book come to fruition.

Priscilla Ebersole, PhD, RN, FAAN

1
Introduction

Ann Schmidt Luggen and Sue E. Meiner

The term *arthritis* originates from a Greek word for joint or *arthron*, and the ending letters of *itis* for inflammation. However, arthritis means more than joint inflammation; it can be represented by swelling, tenderness and/or pain, and even immobility. For millions of Americans, performing everyday activities can be a challenge due to the chronic nature of arthritis in one or more of its many forms. The universality of arthritis poses more disability for some older adults than for others. This variation in signs and symptoms with flare-ups or chronicity often creates difficulties for the primary care provider as well as the patient. Information is needed on specific forms of arthritis with supportive data to provide options of care and treatment to older adults with arthritis.

The toll of degenerative arthritic and rheumatic disorders on older adults can lead to mild, moderate, or severe disability. Joints and connective tissues fail to function smoothly. As the disease progression continues, other conditions such as chronic pain, immobility, poor body image, isolation, and depression can build.

The management of care for the older adult diagnosed with arthritis begins with pain control and promotion of comfort. If inflammation is present, reduction of swelling and the inflammatory process is needed. Balancing daily activities to promote an optimal lifestyle while limiting the damage to affected parts of the body is a major goal of care.

Historical perspectives and demographics will provide a background on the need for understanding the management and care issues of older adults with arthritis. The ultimate goal of management and care is to help older adults achieve the highest quality of life for their remaining life spans.

HISTORY OF ARTHRITIS

Arthritis has been present in man and animals for nearly 100 million years. An arthritis timeline (Wilder, 2000) reveals that iguanadons in Brussels in 85,000,000 BC had primary and secondary osteoarthritis (OA). Neanderthal man (30,000 BC) remains show that early man had secondary OA. In 4500 BC, American Indians in Tennessee had rheumatoid arthritis (RA), the first evidence of this disease. The book of Job (Job 30:16–17) reveals "and the days of affliction have taken hold upon me. My bones are pierced in me in the night season, and my sinews take no rest." The derivative of aspirin, ground willow bark, was known in 500 BC. Hippocrates (400 BC) discussed joint ailments including gout. Julius Caesar (43 BC) had arthritis. Botticellís masterpiece, *Birth of Venus*, reveals that the model probably had arthritis if one closely examines her fingers in the painting. In the 1940's, our soldiers in the tropics noted that quinine and the synthetic chloroquine decreased arthritis symptoms. In 1949, cortisone was first used for RA. In 1977, a genetic marker associated with RA was found. In 1997–1999, new drugs were approved by the Federal Drug Administration (FDA) for treatment of OA and RA, disease-modifying antirheumatic drugs, biologics that inhibit RA inflammation and tissue damage. The new Cox-2 inhibitors, recently approved by the FDA, are nonsteroidal anti-inflammatory drugs (NSAIDs) that are less damaging to the gastric lining compared to other NSAIDs.

On the horizon are disease-modifying anti-OA drugs and a probable increase in the use of alternative medications. A recent survey of an outpatient clinic serving geriatric and rheumatology (arthritis) patients found that the prevalence of use of alternative medications was 66% (Beers & Berkow, 2000). In other countries, rheumatology patients have an increased prevalence of use of alternative medications: 63–91% in Canada, 65–83% in Mexico, 40–99% in Australia, and 81% in Ireland. The National Center for Complementary and Alternative Medicine, a new division in the National Institutes of Health (NIH) was established in 1998 to develop studies of alternative medications for use in medical care.

MUSCULOSKELETAL DISORDERS OF OLDER ADULTS

There are more than 100 different forms of arthritis. Many are very rare, but many are prevalent in older adults. Some of the musculoskeletal disorders that occur in elderly people include OA, RA, osteoporosis (OP), Paget's disease of bone, gout, pseudogout, polymyalgia rheumatica (PMR), idiopathic skeletal hyperostosis, septic arthritis, bursitis, rotator cuff tears, drug-induced systemic lupus erythematosis, and Sjogren's syndrome (Beers & Berkow, 2000). There are others, such as the musculoskeletal disorders of thyroid disease, and polymyositis, which are more common in older rather than younger patients, but are too rare to be discussed in this book.

ARTHRITIS AND DISABILITY

Arthritis is the most commonly reported chronic condition (Beers & Berkow, 2000). It progresses as a disease process with aging. Disability from arthritis greatly affects function, independence, and the need for additional resources or even long term care. In an assessment of older adults with arthritis, the practitioner would want to assess activities of daily living (ADLs) such as ability to eat, bathe, and use the toilet independently, and IADLs, instrumental activities of daily living, such as using the telephone, taking medications as instructed, and doing housework independently. About 5–8% of community elders older than 65 need assistance with one or more ADLs. These needs grow with aging (Beers & Berkow, 2000). Co-morbidity is increasingly prevalent with advancing age, which further increases disability.

TABLE 1.1 Living Arrangements of Older Adults Living Alone

Males		Females	
65–74	14.6%	65–74	32.1%
75–84	19.6%	75–84	50.0%
≥85	29.2%	≥85	58.6%
	Living with spouse		
65–74	76.8%	65–74	51%
75–84	68.2%	75–84	31.5%
≥85	46.%	≥85	10.7%

Adapted from Beers & Berkow, 2000.

Living Arrangements

The living arrangements of community-dwelling older adults >65 are such that as one ages, there is an increased chance that one will live alone (Table 1.1). This information becomes very important in caring for older adults with arthritis and disability in terms of the supports that need to be instituted. Sixty percent of older women 75–84 are widowed.

Sex Demographics for Rheumatic Diseases

Males and females have different musculoskeletal problems. Men are more likely to seek treatment for strain and sprains; women seek treatment for OA (Tosi, 2001). The incidence of *femur neck fracture* is four times greater in females than males. Frozen shoulder (adhesive capsulitis) occurs in 2% of the general population but 75% are in women and 1/3 of these develop it in the other shoulder (Hannafin & Chiara, 2001). Osteoporosis occurs six times more commonly in women and is related to estrogen deficiency in Type I rather than calcium intake (Land, Russel & Kahn, 2000). Type II osteoporosis occurs two times more frequently in women and is associated with hip fracture and lifelong decreased intake of calcium.

Mortality

Older women live longer, live alone, and more often live in poverty and have fewer resources for managing a life with disability (Beers & Berkow, 2000). Nursing home populations are predominantly composed of elderly women.

Poverty

Poverty rates for the elderly are at a new low (1999) with one in every twelve elderly whites reported at poverty level (Administration on Aging, 2000a). Twenty-two percent of older African Americans and 20.4% of elderly Hispanics were at poverty level. Those who live in cities have higher than average poverty rates (11.7%) as do those who live in rural areas. Elders who live in the South have higher than average poverty rates. Older women have higher poverty rates (11.8%) than do older men (6.9%). Those who live alone (mainly older women) are poorer (20.2%) than those who live with their family (5.7%). The highest poverty rate is among Hispanic women who live alone (58.8%). These statistics reveal a tremendous disparity of resources by ethnicity and by sex.

Racial Diversity

Racial diversity is increasingly changing in the U.S. in general and the older population is no exception (Beers & Berkow, 2000). Black and white older adults in the U.S. increased 20% from 1980 to 1990. Hispanic older adults increased 57% and Asian numbers increased 150%. In 1994, 11% of the elderly population of the U.S. were non-white or Hispanic. This is expected to increase to 31% by 2040.

PHYSIOLOGICAL CHANGES OF THE MUSCULOSKELETAL SYSTEM WITH AGING

The following physiological changes that occur with age have an impact on the effect of arthritis in the elderly body:

Bone Density

There is a progressive diminution of bone density beginning at about age 50, which is increased in women. This results in increased deterioration of the microarchitecture of the skeleton with resultant bone fragility and increased risk of fracture. This process is increased by

- Glucocorticoids
- Thyroxine

- Increased alcohol intake
- Immobilization
- Gastrointestinal disorders
- Hypercalciuria
- Cigarette smoking
- Malignancies

Cartilage

There are age-related changes in cartilage such as increased crystallization and calcification, increased chondrocalcinosis, and diminished knee cartilage thickness (Beers & Berkow, 2000).

Connective Tissue

Diminished fibroblast activity results in decreased healing capacity with increasing age. There is a decrease in tensile strength and an increase in stiffness of connective tissue. Ligaments and tendons also decrease in strength.

Muscles

Lean body mass decreases primarily due to a decrease in muscle mass and in the number and size of the muscles. This is sarcopenia. It may be related to decreased physical activity and decrease in protein intake. Age-related loss of muscle fibers is 50% by age 80. Deconditioning occurs rapidly in older adults. Estimates are that with one day of total bed rest, two weeks of reconditioning are needed to return to baseline (Beers & Berkow, 2000).

HEALTHY PEOPLE 2010

Healthy People 2010 is a statement of national health objectives developed by a consortium of agencies and organizations under the auspices of the U.S. Office of Disease Prevention and Health Promotion. It builds on a prevention initiative pursued over the past 20 years. These national health objectives serve as a basis for health planning (U.S. Department of Health and Human Services, 2000). Relevant HP2010 goals are

(1) Increased quality and years of healthy life, and (2) Elimination of health disparities. Focus areas of HP2010 include

- access to health services
- arthritis, osteoporosis, chronic back conditions
- disability and secondary conditions
- education and community-based programs
- physical activity and fitness

It is the goal of this book to build on these initiatives by giving nurses who care for older adults with arthritis the knowledge and the tools they need to assist patients in increasing the quality and years of healthy life without pain and disability.

SUMMARY

Arthritis is a group of diseases that affect older adults in multiple forms. When untreated, it can lead to disability and death in some people and yet cause only mild aches and stiffness in others. Arthritis has been present for millions of years and while progress in understanding the diseases has been made, especially in recent years, in most cases we do not understand why people do or do not get arthritis.

The diagnosis of any of the forms of arthritis crosses age, gender, race/ethnicity, and socioeconomic levels. The effects can change the living arrangements, social contacts, leisure time activities, and basic activities of living for many older adults. The Healthy People 2010 goals specifically address the need for additional research, mutual planning of care and treatment, and implementation of treatment plans for arthritis, osteoporosis, and chronic back conditions. With these goals before us, this handbook aims to share the present management and care of older adults with arthritis.

REFERENCES

Administration on Aging. (2000). *Profiles of older americans.* http://www.aoa.dhhs.gov/stats

Pharmacotherapeutics. 20(8):958–966. www.medscape.com/pp/pharmaco-therapeutics

Beers, M. H. & Berkow, R. (Eds.). (2000). *Merck manual of geriatrics* (3rd ed.). West Point, PA: Merck.

Land, J. M., Russel, L., & Kahn. S. N. (2000). Osteoporosis. *Clinical Orthopedics.*

Tosi, L. L. (2001, March 16).*Clinical Orthopedics.*

U.S. Dept. of Health and Human Services. (2000). *Healthy people 2010.* http://www.health.gov/healthypeople/

Wilder, S. (2000, Jan/Feb). Through the years: An arthritis timeline. *Arthritis Today.*

PART I
Arthritic Diseases and Related Conditions

2

Osteoarthritis

Patricia Birchfield

Osteoarthritis (OA) is a nearly universal, slowly progressing, degenerative condition that affects both men and women as they age. OA of the hip and knee are two of the most important causes of pain and physical disability in adults. In the United States OA is the second most common form of disability, and although it affects men and women equally in later life, women are more likely to be symptomatic (Kee, 2000; Puppione, Schumann, 1999). It is estimated that between 70% and 85% of persons over 55 years of age are afflicted with OA.

OA of the knee has been estimated to affect approximately 6% of the U. S. population and hip OA is estimated to affect 3%. Radiographic evidence, which appears later in the course of the disease, develops in older individuals at the rate of 1% to 2% per year, more in women than in men (Kee, 2000; Townes, 1999). Structural changes visible on radiography include narrowing of the joint space, osteophyte formation, and remodeling of bone around the joints. Because there are no nerve fibers in articular cartilage no symptoms are evident early in the course of OA. With progression of OA multiple sources of pain appear. Periostal irritation as a result of bone modeling, denuded bone, compression of soft tissue by osteophytes, microfractures of subchondral bone, stress on ligaments, synovitis, effusion, and spasm of surrounding muscle all contribute to OA pain (Townes, 1999).

Because OA is so common, health care utilization is very high. Not only are costs incurred due to disability but also to hip and knee replacements and lost days from work, accounting for more than half of the estimated total costs of $15.5 billion dollars due to OA (Kee, 2000).

Primary OA is the most common form of OA and has no known cause; it is often linked to the aging process as well as to family history. Primary OA most often affects the distal interphalangeal joints (DIPs) and can affect the proximal interphalangeal joints (PIPs), although this is not as common. In addition, the hips and knees are often affected and both the cervical and lumbar spine may also be affected (Hart, Doyle, Spector, 1999).

Secondary OA may occur in any of the body's joints as a result of accident or injury including repetitive joint injury, fracture, obesity, or metabolic disease, and can occur at any age (Birchfield, 2000; Cheng, et al., 2000). It may also be found in individuals with hypertension, hypercholesterolemia, and elevated serum glucose. These findings suggest that secondary OA may have systemic and metabolic components in its etiology (Hart, et al., 1999).

EPIDEMIOLOGY

Although osteoarthritis has no known cause the overall incidence and prevalence appear to increase with age. It is thought to result from a complex variety of individual specific characteristics such as immunologic, biomechanical, and inflammatory variables. Functional characteristics such as trauma, joint use, and stressors to joints, such as obesity, are also implicated in OA's etiology (Cardone, & Tallia, A. F., 1999). Age and female gender are generally considered the most important risk factors for the development of OA. Men and women as they age believe that OA is inevitable and that they must learn to accept it. This is not true and the advances that have been made in understanding the pathophysiology of OA are helping to dispel this myth (Birchfield, 2000; Cardone, & Tallia, 1999; Townes, A. S., 1999).

RISK FACTORS IN OSTEOARTHRITIS

Nutrition

Obesity is an obvious risk factor for the development of OA and is more often associated with progressive OA of the knee than of the hip (Birchfield, 2000; Cardone, & Tallia, 1999). The most obvious explanation is that obesity places individuals at a mechanical disadvantage as greater muscle power is required for daily activities. Even in individuals who do not have OA, obesity has been shown to be associated with voluntary weakness of the quadriceps muscle (Creamer, Lethridge, & Hochberg, 2000). A widespread assumption is that the link between obesity and OA has to do with the repetition of greater axial load; however this does not explain the difference in prevalence among the lower joints. The relationship between obesity and hip OA reveals that the load on the hip with excess weight is substantially lower than the load on the knee. Even a small loss of weight can slow progression and show improvement in knee OA (Kee, 2000).

Hormonal Influences

The increased prevalence of OA in women and the progression of the disease after menopause suggest the possibility of hormonal influence. Before age 50 the incidence of OA is greater in men but that changes after women turn 50. This change suggests that loss of estrogen may be a risk factor (Kee, 2000).

Estrogen has many complex conflicting effects that may affect cartilage repair and degradation. Estrogen prevents the activation of osteoclasts and the resulting bone loss that follows. Bony attrition is seen in late stages of OA and it may be that estrogen helps stabilize joints by preventing bone loss and thus may also preserve bone density. High bone density has been linked to OA. Conversely, less bone density could mean more joint tolerance to forceful impact, resulting in less cartilage damage (Editorial, 1999, Kee, 2000). More study is needed for definitive answers to the questions of effects of estrogen on OA.

Genetics and Family History

OA is considered to be a group of clinically heterogenous disorders. Although the etiology of OA is unknown there is evidence to support the importance of genetic factors in some subgroups of OA, especially in hand and knee OA (Huang, Ushiyama, Kawasaki, & Hukuda, 2000). Although genetic factors most likely involve multiple genes, specific gene mutations resulting in changes of joint components lead to the development of OA have been described (Cardone, & Tallia, 1999).

It has been noted that there is a preponderance of OA in women and it has been suggested that genetic susceptibility may be greater in women than in men. Hereditary abnormalities in structural components of cartilage are also implicated in the development of OA (Mustafa, et al., 2000). As the molecular revolution continues to progress, more genes will be found to play a role in the development of OA. However, more research on the complex interaction among genetics, family history, and environment is needed.

Activity

One of the best determinants of bone mineral density (BMD) is activity level. Some forms of exercise can increase bone density in specific areas of the body. BMD can increase up to 26% in some areas by loading the skeleton through physical exercise (Sharkey, Williams, & Guerin, 2000). Strenuous, high intensity, and repetitive exercise, both sport and occupational, has been associated with the development of OA, although there appears to be no increased evidence of OA with recreational exercise (Kee, 2000).

Cartilage is an avascular tissue that depends on diffusion of substances through the cartilage matrix from joint fluid for nourishment of mature cartilage cells. The loading and physical activity induced by everyday activities produces pressure gradients and fluid flows into the tissue that enhances the process (Sharkey, et al., 2000).

Normal loads on joints can accelerate degeneration in an already deformed, unconstrained, or damaged joint. High impact loading, by virtue of either single or repetitive events, may lead to joint degeneration. Ignoring joint trauma and continuing to exercise the affected joint is a known risk factor for the development of OA. Too little loading may be harmful also as disuse has been found to have adverse, although reversible, effects on cartilage (Sharkey, et al., 2000). Some studies have found no conclusive evidence for or against exercise; these findings bear watching, especially because of the known beneficial cardiovascular effects of exercise (Sharma, Lou, Cahue, & Dunlop, 2000).

Exercise in later life should be encouraged to increase strength, co-ordination, and balance, thus reducing the likelihood of falls. One of the most important outcomes of regular exercise in older individuals is an improvement in, or preservation of, functional independence which is associated with decreased mortality (Sharkey, et al., 2000).

Loss of Muscle

Loss of muscle (sarcopenia) in older persons may also be a contrib-uting factor in either the development or progression of OA. A diag-nosis of OA leads to atrophy proximal to the involved joint as a result of progressive weakness and disuse. The loss of supporting muscle may increase the joint load, which can then lead to cartilage damage, especially in the weight-bearing joints of the body. Resis-tance exercise and muscle strengthening may decrease knee symp-toms (Kee, 2000).

Occupation

Work-related activities, thought to be due to repeated minor trauma, have been linked to the development of OA. Repeated minor trauma may exacerbate an already increased risk of a joint that is predis-posed due to an underlying mechanical factor such as malalignment or deformity (Cardone & Tallia, 1999).

Older individuals who garden and/or walk may have an increased risk of OA, cotton mill workers have a higher incidence of Heber-dens' nodes (arthritis symptoms on hands), and those who perform duties that require crouching or kneeling may have a higher inci-dence of knee OA (Kee, 2000).

Trauma

A history of prior trauma may be an important risk factor for the development of OA in a joint damaged by ligamentous instability or meniscal tear in the knee. Prior surgery is also a risk factor in the development of OA. Repetitive stress and minor injury may predis-pose a person to OA and may account for sites where OA has been found that are not commonly affected, such as elbows in baseball pitchers and upper limb OA in hammer operators (Townes, 1999).

Pathology

The human body has three types of joints (see Table 2.1): diarthroidal, or synovium lined joints, which are involved in the movement of limbs; synarthrosis or pseudo joints; and amphiarthroses, or cartilaginous joints. In OA the diarthroidal joints are affected; these include joints of the hand, hip, and knee (Cardone & Tallia, 1999).

OA is characterized by degeneration of the joint cartilage which results in the formation of new bone at the articular, or joint, margins. This joint degeneration and the resulting formation of new bone results in pain and stiffness of the joints that are affected. All of the diarthroidal joints can be affected but OA is seen most commonly in the hands, hips, and knees (O'Rourke, 2001). The properties of articular cartilage are the core of OA pathology. Articular cartilage is composed of water, proteoglycans, chondrocytes, and other matrix components. The functional properties of cartilage result from the unique structure of chondrocytes, which are embedded in a matrix of collagen and proteoglycan. Proteoglycans, which have a half life of three months, are responsible for the porous structure of cartilage, trapping and holding water (O'Rourke, 2001).

Proteoglycan and type II collagen are two of the major components of articular cartilage. Type II collagen makes up 90% to 95% of the total collagen content and allows for a cartilaginous framework and tensile strength. Proteoglycans are protein polysaccharides and are responsible for the compressive strength of cartilage. Proteoglycans are produced by chondrocytes, which in aging become hypocelluar and larger, and no longer reproduce. With the loss of chondrocytes, cartilage becomes stiff and hypocellular, and decreas-

TABLE 2.1 Joints of the Body With Examples

Joints of the Body	Examples
Diarthroidal (synovium lined)	Sacroiliac, shoulder, hip, interphalangeal
Synarthrosis (pseudo joints)	Skull, bodies of vertebrae
Amphiarthroses (cartilaginous)	symphysis pubis, manibriosternal (sternum)

es in solubility. Cartilage proteoglycans decrease in size and mass. Also, protein content increases and water content decreases, causing a decrease in cartilage elasticity.

With time, the catabolism of proteoglycans and loss of chondrocytes result in abrasion of cartilage and the formation of new bone within the joint. With healthy individuals, a balance of cartilage turnover exists through synthesis and degradation. One possible explanation for the development of OA is failure to maintain this homeostasis (O'Rourke, 2001). Another theory suggests that subchondral bone may sustain repeated microfractures that result in stiffening and ineffective shock absorbing. Subchondral bone changes are viewed as an important cause of OA rather than a sequel of cartilage damage (O'Rourke, 2001).

Most OA presents as monoarticular disease but it may present as polyarticular in the load-bearing joints, especially the knees, hips, and vertebral joints (Sharkey, et al., 2000). Changes in the load-bearing joints are most pronounced on the articular cartilage. Susceptibility to cartilage damage increases with age and may be the result of abnormal biomechanics that lead to stress and alteration in the normal structure. Compensatory attempts at bone repair result in remodeling at the ends of bones with osteophyte formation. Early in the course of the disease synovitis is minimal but as OA progresses it may contribute to joint damage (Kee, 2000; Townes, 1999).

CLINICAL FEATURES

Pain is the most commonly reported complaint in OA. Early in the course of the disease individuals may report poorly localized, asymmetric, and intermittent pain that is aching and nagging in quality. Pain usually occurs with movement and is relieved with rest. In advanced cases of the disease, the individual may be kept awake during the night because of pain. Pain may be referred, such as cervical OA being reported as shoulder and/or neck pain. Hip OA may be reported as pain in the medial aspect of the thigh. More severe reports of pain are usually localized to the affected joint (Cardone & Tallia, 1999; Townes, 1999).

Stiffness in affected joints is also a very common complaint. Early in the course of the disease stiffness is experienced after a period of rest when activity is resumed. Later, it may become a persistent and bothersome complaint. Morning stiffness generally lasts no more than 30 minutes. As the disease progresses, particles of degenerated cartilage may shed into the joint; this produces loose bodies that may cause the joint to lock or give way (Birchfield, 2000; Puppione, & Schumann, 1999; Townes, 1999).

Inflammation, swelling, crepitus, synovitis, and joint effusion may also be present. Heberden's nodes, and less commonly Bouchard's nodes, if present on the DIPs and PIPs respectively, are painful at first but subside over time leaving joint deformity and limitation of movement (Kee, 2000; Sharkey, 2000). Tenderness to palpation over the joint is common but may be mild or absent. Inflammation, swelling, and joint effusion are seen more often in more advanced cases of OA. Knees are more likely to experience effusion and generally do not reveal any warmth or erythema. Joint mobility may be limited, leading to joint deformities; again this occurs later in the course of OA. When the knee and/or hip is involved, gait may be impaired, leaving the individual with a noticeable limp (Townes, 1999).

DIAGNOSIS

There is no definitive laboratory test to aid in the diagnosis of OA; it is a diagnosis that is made clinically. Normal lab values, unless there is another coexisting disease state, are seen in OA. If there is inflammation the erythrocyte sedimentation rate (ESR) may be elevated. Tests for rheumatoid factor or antinuclear antibodies may be normally elevated in older adults. C-reactive protein may also reveal mild elevations and increased levels may predict progression of OA (Kee, 2000; Townes, 1999). Joint aspiration may be performed as a method to eliminate other diagnoses when effusion is present. Synovial fluid in OA is usually of the noninflammatory type, with normal viscosity, few leukocytes, and a normal differential count (Cardone & Tallia, 1999; Townes, 1999).

One of the key features of OA is the lack of association between joint pain and joint deformity on radiography early in the course of the disease. Radiographic joint changes may reveal varied signs and symptoms of pain and disability. These changes may be seen and yet the individual may be asymptomatic; however, this is not usually the case. The more OA progresses the more likely changes will become visible on radiography. Typical changes seen on radiography include joint space narrowing, sclerosis of the subchondral bone, bony cysts, osteophytes, and evidence of joint deformity (Kee, 2000; Sharkey, et al., 2000).

MANAGEMENT

Treatment modalities for OA focus on primary and secondary prevention. Primary prevention involves education regarding joint protection, exercise, weight reduction, and avoidance of repetitive motion. Secondary prevention is primarily palliative, involving both pharmacological and nonpharmacological measures. Occupational and physical therapy, aerobic and muscle strengthening exercise, assistive devices, appropriate shoes, and use of orthotics to correct abnormal biomechanics are often utilized as forms of nonpharmacologic treatment (O'Rourke, 2001). Although acetaminophen is considered the drug of choice in OA, other agents such as capsaicin, methylsalicylate, COX-2 inhibitors, nonsteroidal anti-inflammatory drugs (NSAIDs), corticosteroids, hyalruonan, and rarely opiates may be utilized as well. None of these drugs control the progression of OA (O'Rourke, 2001).

Even though OA affects millions of adults there are currently no curative treatments for this disease. Even more important, there is no evidence to support that any treatment alters the course of the disease. Thus, treatment is supportive and symptomatic and centered around keeping persons active. The primary goals of treatment are to relieve pain, maintain joint function and mobility, and reduce joint swelling. The optimal treatment involves a combined approach focusing on modifications of risk factors, particular obesity, and specific treatments such as exercise and pharmacotherapy (Puppione, & Schumann, 1999).

A collaborative approach among nursing, medicine, and physical and occupational therapy may help individuals reduce disability and maintain function. Collaborative management of OA assists in providing individualized and effective care. This approach to care and symptom management will keep individuals functional longer and may reduce the need for surgery (Puppione, Schumann, 1999).

PHARMACOTHERAPY

NSAIDs

For a long time, NSAIDs have been the mainstay of drug therapy in OA. Because of their effect on the gastrointestinal mucosa and kidneys, these drugs add an increased risk of potentially serious side effects, especially with long-term use. Acetaminophen in doses of up to 4000 mg daily may be taken to control pain if liver function tests are and remain within normal limits. Individuals with advanced disease or who have no relief with acetaminophen may respond better to NSAIDs (Cardone & Tallia, 1999; Townes, 1999).

The clinical effects of NSAIDs result primarily from the inhibition of the enzyme cyclooxygenase (COX), the first step in the process of converting arachidonic acid to prostaglandins (Day, et al., 2000). The newer drugs on the market are referred to as COX-2 inhibitor drugs. COX-1 helps to protect the stomach and prevent ulcers. COX-2 inhibitors relieve pain but because they do not inhibit COX-1, as NSAIDs do, the gastrointestinal tract is protected.

Celebrex® (Celecoxib) cannot be given if an individual is allergic to sulfa drugs but Vioxx® (Rofecoxib) can. Neither drug should be given if a person is allergic to aspirin and they should not be given along with an NSAID (Kee, 2001). Both the Celecoxib Long-Term Arthritis Safety Study (CLASS) and the Vioxx® Gastrointestinal Outcomes Research (VIGOR) trials found that there were fewer incidences of gastrointestinal side effects with COX-2 inhibitor medications. These findings have led the American College of Rheumatology to recommend utilizing these drugs in the treatment of OA of the hip and knee at recommended dosages. COX-2 inhibitor medications can cause renal toxicity, so caution must be exercised if individuals have hypertension, heart failure, or mild to moderate renal insufficiency. Neither should be used in cases of severe renal insufficiency (Altman & Hochberg, 2001). The subjects in the VIGOR study, who were not on concomitant aspirin as many in the CLASS study were, revealed that patients treated with a non COX-2 inhibitor NSAID had fewer incidents of stroke or cardiac deaths. The explanation for this is unknown but might represent the anti-platelet effect of the other NSAID. OA is common in older individuals, many of whom may have cardiac comorbidities; however, the effect of taking rofecoxib with aspirin is unknown and further study is needed to fully understand the implications (Altman & Hochberg, 2001).

Intra-articular injections of suspension of corticosteroids are effective for most people with pain relief lasting for weeks and sometimes months. High or repeated doses of corticosteroids may impede the repair process of cartilage, however, and should not be given more than every three months. Recently, hyaluronan has been approved for individuals with OA. This drug is a naturally occurring substance found in synovial fluid and cartilage (Huskisson & Donnelly, 1999). It is given in a series of three to five injections into the knee joint. The injections are viscous and are intended to substitute for hyaluronic acid normally found in the joint (Kee, 2000; Cardone & Tallia, 1999).

Glucosamine

Chondroprotective or disease-modifying antirheumatic drugs (DMARDs) may assist in joint repair and preservation of joint structure and function. Glucosamine is a natural compound that is found in almost all human tissue, especially cartilaginous tissue, and is readily incorporated into proteoglycan molecules. Glucosamine has not been classified as a DMARD for OA; rather it has been characterized as a slow-acting drug for OA. Experimental evidence in vitro suggests that glucosamine may benefit cartilage metabolic processes (O'Rourke, 2001).

Glucosamine's effects are anti-inflammatory in nature and appear to be related to mechanisms that are very different from those of NSAIDs, which act primarily through the inhibition of cyclooxygenases. Glucosamine's action may be related to stimulation of proteoglycan biosynthesis. Newly synthesized proteoglycans are thought to stabilize cell membranes, which results in anti-inflammatory benefits (O'Rourke, 2001).

Chondroitin Sulfate

Chondroitin sulfate is similar to glucosamine, has anti-inflammatory effects, and affects cartilage metabolism. Glucosamine has a 90% absorption rate in the gastrointestinal tract whereas chondroitin sulfate has only a 10% rate. It is thought that the addition of chondroitin sulfate assists in proteoglycan concentration and a decrease in collagenlytic activity. A cautious and slow course of treatment is advised for both glucosamine and chondroitin as there are no federal standards to regulate strength and purity (O'Rourke, 2001).

NURSING MANAGEMENT

General health promotion measures are advisable for all individuals but are especially crucial to aging persons. Health promotion measures may help in delaying the onset and progression of OA. Although age, gender, and family history are not amenable to intervention, other factors are (Kee, 2000).

The following nursing diagnoses are appropriate for the older patient with OA:

- Altered nutrition, more than body requirements, related to decreased activity from pain
- Pain, chronic pain related to arthritis disease process
- Risk for injury from overuse of joints
- Risk for disuse of joints related to pain

Interventions and Outcomes

Altered nutrition, more than body requirements, related to decreased activity from pain

Expected outcome: The patient will lose weight after changing diet and increasing exercise.

Nursing Interventions

Promote an exercise program.

Exercise is recognized as an important part of successful aging in spite of conflicting reports about the benefits and risks of exercise in individuals with OA. If there are fears of exercise with the accompanying potential for injury, these must be addressed prior to initiating an exercise program to improve compliance. The goals of an exercise program for persons with OA include pain reduction, increasing range of motion and muscle strength, improving balance and coordination, and prevention of disability and poor health from inactivity (Cardone & Tallia, 1999; Kee, 2000; Puppione & Schumann, 1999; Sharkey, et al., 2000). Because along with aging, OA results in increased muscle and joint stiffness and reduced tissue elasticity, any exercise session should begin with a warm-up and stretching component. Gradual conditioning is essential in order not to aggravate muscle pain. If pain is worse after exercise the intensity should be reduced or halted until the symptoms have subsided. Low impact exercises, such as walking three times per week for at least 30 minutes, is a reasonable target for most people. Supervised fitness walking with light stretching and strengthening exercises improves pain and physical fitness while reducing the need for medication (Sharkey, 2000; Townes, 1999).

Support the patient's efforts to lose weight.

Weight reduction activities, for those individuals in whom it is needed, is very important in any treatment plan. Even a small weight loss can result in immediate and recognizable positive effects. Anyone undertaking a weight loss regimen should be cautioned against food fads as these could be potentially harmful. A possible association between low serum levels of vitamins C and D in the progression of OA indicates that an adequate dietary intake of these vitamins is also an important consideration (Townes, 1999).

Pain, chronic pain related to arthritis disease process

Expected outcome: Patient will state that the pain is manageable and there is greater comfort.

Nursing Interventions

Teach the patient about around-the-clock pain medications for improved sleeping and increased ability to exercise. Assess pain and pain relief regularly. Recommend stronger analgesics such as narcotics in end-stage or very severe arthritis. Teach about alternatives to medication for pain relief. Moist heat is preferable to dry heat for the relief of pain. Superficial heat treatments do not generally penetrate into deeper tissues. Deep heat, such as ultrasound, can be beneficial in relieving pain. Cold is recommended after exercise as a method to reduce pain and muscle spasms (Cardone & Tallia, 1999).

Discuss assistive devices and rest. Rest from weight bearing and stability when walking may be partially achieved by the use of a crutch, cane, walker, or splint. How the individual feels about such devices is important to consider because many will feel that these aids are visible signs of infirmity and refuse to utilize them (Kee, 2000; Townes, 1999).

Risk for injury from overuse of joints

Expected outcomes: The patient will not suffer new injuries and will be able to discuss the need for rest and exercise.

Nursing Interventions

Teach about non-weight-bearing exercises. Suggest ways to rest during activities, such as sitting in a chair when doing kitchen activities and meal preparation, rather than standing. Pain and the discomfort of OA may be exacerbated by weight bearing and may accelerate cartilage destruction. Therefore, rest is also an important treatment measure for OA. Short periods of rest throughout the day are more effective than longer and less frequent periods of rest (Townes, 1999).

Risk for disuse of joints related to pain

Expected outcome: The patient will state the importance of joint use, the effects of non-use and the need to maintain range of motion.

Nursing Intervention

Instruct the patient about loss of strength and mobility with disuse. Maintenance of quadricep strength is particularly important in OA of the knee. This can be accomplished by beginning a full slow extension of the knee against gravity and then, as progress allows, by slowly adding increasing amounts of weight to the lower leg. Once the knee is extended, the quadriceps should be tightened and held for 10 to 15 seconds. Other aerobic exercises that can be recommended for persons with OA include cycling, swimming, and aerobic pool exercises (Cardone & Tallia, 1999).

COMPLEMENTARY THERAPIES

Acupuncture and therapeutic touch have also been explored as an adjunct to the treatment of individuals with OA. Acupuncture was performed on older individuals over a 4-, 8-, and 12-week period. Improvement was noted at the 8-week interval after acupuncture had been delivered biweekly along with conventional treatment. Some decay in the benefits of acupuncture was noted at the 12-week interval, although there was still substantial improvement over baseline (Berman, et al., 1999) Merenstein and D'Amico (1999) found that therapeutic touch can relieve the pain and improve the level of functioning in individuals with OA of at least one knee who do not have connective tissue disease.

SUMMARY AND CONCLUSION

Osteoarthritis is one of the most prevalent conditions of aging, and with the number of aging individuals rising, the incidence and prevalence can do nothing but rise as well. Because the etiology of OA is unknown, so also is its prevention and treatment. However, developing recognition of predisposing risk factors and pathophysiology suggests prudent steps that can be recommended, such as weight loss, physical conditioning and muscle strengthening exercises, avoiding repetitive stress and injury to a joint, and maintenance of good nutrition (Townes, 1999).

Even though there are no known cures, there are potentially effective interventions. Education is a primary component of any treatment plan and is one way of getting the individual involved in self care. Complementary therapies should be discussed to allow for flexibility in self care as well as to discover any potential interactions with other treatment modalities (Kee, 2000).

Any treatment plan should always include health promotion activities, which are crucial to individuals as they age. These activities are aimed at relieving pain, maintaining joint stability, and reducing associated symptoms such as joint swelling and effusion (Puppione & Schumann, 1999). Osteoarthritis can be effectively managed through vigilance and attention to therapeutic regimens, as well as to new research findings.

REFERENCES

Altman, R. D., & Hochberg, M. C. (2001, June 30.) Do COX-2 inhibitors offer reduced GI toxicity? *Patient Care*, 12–27.

Berman, B. M., Singh, B. B., Langenberg, L. P., Hadhazy, L. V., Bareta, J., & Hochberg, M. (1999). A randomized trial of acupuncture as an adjunctive therapy in osteoarthritis of the knee. *British Society for Rheumatology, 38*, 346–354.

Birchfield, P. C. (2000). Arthritis: Osteoarthritis and rheumatoid arthritis. In D. Robinson, K. Rogers, & P. Kidd (Eds.), *Primary care across the lifespan* (pp. 89–95). St. Louis: Mosby.

Cardone, D. A., & Tallia, A. F. (1999). Osteoarthritis. In J. K. Singleton, S. A. Sandowski, C. Green-Hernandez, T. V. Horvath, R. V. Di Gregorio, S. R. Holzemer (Eds.), *Primary care* (pp. 543–548). Philadelphia: Lippincott.

Cheng, Y., Macera, C. A., Davis, D. R., Ainsworth, B. E., Troped, P. J., & Blair, S. N. (2000). Physical activity and self-reported, physician diagnosed osteoarthritis: Is physical activity a risk factor? *Journal of Clinical Epidemiology, 3*, 315–322.

Creamer, P., Lethridge, M., & Hochberg, M. C. (2000). Factors associated with functional impairment in symptomatic knee osteoarthritis. *Rheumatology, 39*, 490–496.

Day, R., Morrison, B., Luza, A., Castaneda, O., Strusberg, A., Nahir, M., et al. (2000). A randomized trial of the efficacy and tolerability of the COX-2 inhibitor Rofecoxib vs Ibuprofen in patients with osteoarthritis. *Archives of Internal Medicine, 160*, 1781–1787.

Editorial. (1999). Estrogen and arthritis: How do we explain conflicting study results? *Preventive Medicine, 28*, 445–448.

Hart, D. J., Doyle, D. V., & Spector, T. D. (1999). Incidence and risk factors for radiographic knee osteoarthritis in middle-aged women: The Chingford study. *Arthritis & Rheumatism, 42*, 17–24.

Huang, J., Ushiyama, K. I., Kawaskai, T., & Hukuda, S. (2000). Vitamin D receptor gene polymorphisms and osteoarthritis of the hand, hip, and knee: A case control study in Japan. *Rheumatology, 2,*(39), 79–84.

Huskisson, E. C., & Donnelly, S. (1999). Hyaluronic acid in the treatment of the knee. *Rheumatology, 38*, 602–607.

Kee, C. K. (2000). Osteoarthritis: Manageable scourge of aging. *Rheumatology, 35*, 199–208.

Merenstein, G. A. & D'Amico, J. H. (1999). Therapeutic touch and osteoarthritis of the knee. *Journal of Family Practice, 48*, 11–12.

Mustafa, Z., Chapman, C. I., Carr, A. J., Clipsham, K., Chitnavis, J., Sinsheimer, J. S., Bloomfield, V. A., McCartney, M., Cox, O., Sykes, J. S., & Louhlin, J. (2000). Linkage analysis of candidate genes as susceptibility loci for arthritis-suggestive linkage of COL9A1 to female hip osteoarthritis. *Rheumatology, 39*, 299–306.

O'Rourke, M. (2001). Determining the efficacy of glucosamine and chondroitin for osteoarthritis. *The Nurse Practitioner, 26*, 33–52.

Puppione, A. A. & Schumann, T. (1999). Management strategies for older adults with osteoarthritis: How to promote and maintain function. *Journal of the American Academy of Nurse Practitioners, 11*, 167–171.

Sharkey, N. A., Williams, N. I., & Guerin, J. B. (2000). The role of exercise in the prevention and treatment of osteoporosis and osteoarthritis. *Rheumatology, 35*, 209–212.

Sharma, L. Lou, C., Cahue, S., & Dunlop, D. D. (2000). The mechanism of the effect of obesity in knee osteoarthritis. *Arthritis and Rheumatism, 43*, 568–575.

Townes, A.S. (1999). Osteoarthritis. In L. R. Barker, J. R. Burton, P. D. Zieve, (Eds.). *Principles of ambulatory medicine* (pp. 960–973). Baltimore: Williams & Wilkins.

3
Rheumatoid Arthritis

Ann Schmidt Luggen

Rheumatoid arthritis (RA) is a systemic autoimmune disorder of unknown etiology with chronic, symmetric, erosive synovitis of peripheral joints. There are many extra-articular manifestations affecting mortality. The outcome has been poor because the disease usually starts in middle age and progresses with aging through joint destruction, deformity, and disability, despite appropriate therapy. However, this is an exciting time for the management of RA because there are several new types of medications recently approved by the FDA that may affect the usual course of the disease.

EPIDEMIOLOGY

The prevalence of RA increases with age and occurs in about 1% of the population worldwide and 10% of adults older than 65. The female-to-male ratio is 3:1. The incidence is low in China and high in Pima Indians of the U.S.(Firesteen, 2001). There is no ethnic group unaffected by RA. A study in Finland reveals that the incidence of RA is declining in younger adults, and increasing in older adults (Kaipiainen-seppanen, Aho, Isomaki, & Laakso, 1996) perhaps due to changes in the host-environment relationship. In the Northern hemisphere, the onset of RA occurs more in winter than in summer (Harris, 2001a). It occurs more than twice as often between October and March than during the other months.

RA is classified as seropositive or seronegative. Eighty percent of people with RA are rheumatoid factor antibody positive. This is associated with a more severe, progressive course with earlier onset of joint destruction. Life expectancy is decreased by 10 to 15 years. Older adults clinically diagnosed with RA who are rheumatoid factor negative can later become positive.

There is controversy over whether RA in older adults is a specific clinical subset of RA. Mavragani and Moutsopoulos(1999) describe LORA (late onset RA) which has a late, > 60 years of age of onset, a more equal sex distribution, higher frequency of abrupt onset, more large joint involvement, and fewer extra-articular features than RA in younger adults.

There appears to be an association or increased risk of having RA and developing cancers (Harris, 2001a). RA patients have a two to three times greater risk for developing Hodgkin's disease, non-Hodgkin's lymphoma, and leukemia. The risk of non-Hodgkin's lymphoma occurring in RA patients with Felty's syndrome is 13 times higher than in non-RA adults.

Risk factors and a predisposition to RA appear to be multifactorial, but at this time little is known. There seems to be an accumulation of influences of genetic and environmental factors that are additive in an individual at a particular point in time (Harris, 2001). A known risk factor is a polymorphism in the genes for T cell receptors or for immunoglobulins. A shared epitope on HLA-DRB chains predisposes to severity of disease. The National Institutes of Health (NIH) is currently sponsoring a consortium to collect genetic material to search for genes to link with phenotypes of the disease (Harris, 2001a). The following are some of the suspected risk factors for RA.

- There is an increased risk (8 times higher than normal) for a twin of an individual with RA.
- Oral contraceptives may be protective for severe disease.
- Having more than 3 children may increase the risk of developing severe RA.

- There is increased morbidity and mortality in women with a lower education level.
- In one study of 377,841 female health professionals, women who smoked were at significant risk for RA and seropositive RA.
- There is an association of RA with gout. Seropositive RA patients should be evaluated for hyperuricemia.
- There is no risk for silicone breast implants and RA.
- There is no relationship between diet and RA.
- There seems to be an inverse relationship between atopy and RA, in which those with allergies have a lower incidence of RA (Harris, 2001a).

Prognostic Factors

The following disease factors correlate with a poorer prognosis and greater likelihood of joint destruction (Harris, 2001).

- Positive rheumatoid factor in serum
- Rheumatoid nodules
- Onset in young woman
- Synovial fluid abnormalities, wbc > 50,000/mm3
- Synovial fluid acidosis

There is a 15-year diminished life expectancy for people with RA. Death from heart disease and stroke is accelerated in elders with RA.

PATHOGENESIS/PATHOPHYSIOLOGY

The cause of RA is unknown. Recent work implicates small molecule mediators of inflammation, cytokines, growth factors, chemokines, adhesion molecules, and metalloproteinases as possible causes of RA. They activate cells from peripheral blood that proliferate and activate cells of the synovium. There is then invasion and destruction of articular cartilage, subchondral bone, tendons, and ligaments. This occurs early in RA, which indicates a need to identify the disease RA very early in its course in order to begin therapy.

Multiple factors are implicated in the pathogenesis of RA (Harris, 2001a). There appears to be a genetic predisposition to RA in some patients. Further, the predominance of women with RA suggests a hormonal effect on immune function. Other research reveals an environmental stimulus, a virus or retrovirus persisting even after the absence of the offending agent. Epstein-Barr virus (EBV) is one of those implicated in the pathogenesis of RA (Harris, 2001a).

CLINICAL FEATURES IN OLDER ADULTS

Onset

RA usually begins in middle age; however, it is not rare for onset to occur in old age. The onset may be insidious or may manifest as an acute episode. There seems to be a tendency for an abrupt onset in the older person as well as an increased likelihood of remission compared to younger RA patients. However, some studies have revealed a more severe course in men and in elderly patients (Gordon & Hastings, 1997)

The onset of most cases of RA is slow and insidious, over weeks to months. Early symptoms may be articular or systemic. There may be fatigue, malaise, diffuse musculoskeletal pain, tendon pain, morning stiffness and edema, with painful swollen joints presenting later. It may present asymmetrically with a symmetrical pattern evolving later. Usually, there is symmetrical involvement of joints of hands, wrists, elbows, shoulders, knees, ankles and feet. Any diarthrodial joint can be affected.

Course

The course and complications of chronic RA are complex and variable. Some patients progress from the onset with unrelenting disease activity and systemic features of RA. In most cases, over many years there is slow progression with periods of remission. In some patients the disease may burn out, leaving residual joint damage (Gordon & Hastings, 1997). Joint involvement is symmetrical and wrists, fingers, knees and feet are the most commonly affected (Gordon & Hastings, 1997). Severe disease is associated with large joints with greater amounts of synovium in the knees, elbows, and shoulders. The disease course and examination of articular RA is described by regional areas.

Hands

Typical RA manifests with symmetrical swelling of the metacarpophalangeal (MCP) and proximal interphalangeal (PIP) joints (Gordon & Hastings, 1997). Distal interphalangeal involvement (DIP) may be seen but is probably concomitant OA. Palpation of tenderness will determine disease activity. Ask the client to make a fist, which is difficult with swelling and stiffness, and check grip strength. Look for Raynaud's phenomenon and palmar erythema, which is fairly common. Common late deformities seen in older patients are

- Boutonniere deformity PIP flexion and DIP hyperextension
- Swan-neck deformity MCP flexion, PIP hyperextension, and DIP flexion
- Boutonniere thumb MCP flexion deformity with secondary IP hyperextension
- Flailed thumb-synovitis resulting in destruction of collateral ligaments
- Carpal supination-subluxation of wrist-prominent distal ulna, extensor tendon rupture, contractures, radial erosion with resulting stiffness and/or instability

Elbow

An early sign of involvement is loss of extension. Later, with loss of flexion, the patient has less ability to do self care. Look for effusions that may be palpable in the dimple of the elbow. Swelling can be associated with ulnar entrapment neuropathy or entrapment of the radial nerve. Check for crepitus with pronation and supination. The elbow is a common place for subcutaneous nodules—a cardinal feature of RA. These may break down and form cysts that can easily become infected and lead to systemic infection or septic arthritis.

Shoulder

The shoulder becomes a feature in late stage progressive disease. Symptoms are uncommon until disease/destruction is advanced. Effusions may appear below the acromion. Local bursae may swell and rupture. The long head of the biceps may rupture; this will be seen as a biceps bulge when the client flexes the elbow against resistance. The rotator cuff, a significant site of tears in older adults, is lined with synovium and may be a site of pain and inflammation.

Temporomandibular Joints (TMJs)

These are commonly involved in RA. There is pain, tenderness, and limitation of movement of the jaw when opening the mouth. Over time, there may be a receding jaw.

Cricoarytenoid Joint

This joint is associated with hoarseness. Limitation of its movement may cause aspiration into the lung. Older adults with RA in this area who have a concomitant upper respiratory infection may have a critical upper airway obstruction with stridor, requiring tracheostomy.

Cervical Spine

In severe erosive RA, cervical subluxation in several directions is common. Atlantoaxial subluxation is fairly common. Neurological symptoms do not have a relationship to degree of subluxation, and are probably more related to variations in the diameter of the spinal canal. MRI is valuable in determining pathological anatomy. Early signs of subluxation are

- Pain radiating to the occiput
- Slowly progressive spastic quadriparesis with painless sensory loss in the hands
- Transient episodes of medullary dysfunction with paresthesias in the shoulders or arms during head movement
- Resistance to passive spine motion

Symptoms of spinal cord compression that require intervention include (Harris, 2001).

- Drop attacks
- Changes in level of consciousness
- Peripheral paresthesias without signs of   peripheral nerve disease or compression
- Sensation of the head falling forward on flexion of the cervical spine
- Loss of sphincter control
- Dysphagia, vertigo, convulsions, hemiplegia,   dysarthria, nystagmus

Involvement of the thoracic and lumbar spine is very uncommon in RA. However, compression fractures from the osteoporosis of

RA, aggravated by prednisone therapy, is common in the thoracic region.

Hip

RA involvement in the hip occurs later in the disease process and is subtle. But many clients with longstanding RA have hip involvement. The femoral head may collapse from avascular necrosis and be resorbed and the acetabulum is remodeled and pushed medially so that there is significant protrusion bilaterally. There is loss of internal rotation and stiffness and pain now interfere with the ability to walk (Harris, 2001; Gordon & Hastings, 1997).

Knee

Involvement of the knee in RA is obvious. Small effusions are detectable using the bulge sign. The knee is usually cool compared to other surrounding areas; if it is warm, it may indicate an inflammatory process. When the knee effusion is large, patients assume a fairly constant positioning with the knee flexed and loss of full knee extension occurs. Over time, the knee progresses with disease and there is limitation in walking similar to the disability with the RA hip (Gordon & Hastings, 1997). As cartilage is lost, there is laxity of collateral and cruciate ligaments. Baker's cysts in the popliteal area may extend down to the medial aspect of the calf and occasionally even to the ankle. The cyst arises as an extension (Gordon & Hastings, 1997) from the joint cavity. Exertion may cause rupture and extravasation of inflammatory synovial fluid, presenting a picture that resembles thrombophlebitis.

Foot

Many areas of the foot are involved in RA. The metatarsal heads in the forefoot cause much pain and disability. Synovitis of the metatarsophalangeal (MTP) joints and the flexor tendons cause patients to walk on their heels. This eventually leads to clawing of the toes and eventual dorsal dislocation of the MTP joint. Heel pain can be a particular problem in RA. There may be a bursitis and nodule formation in the Achilles tendon. There may be synovitis in the subtalar and talonavicular joints, which is common in RA. Muscle spasm is common and results in a valgus deformity and spastic flat foot. Pressure points on the head of the talus results and the joint may spontaneously fuse.

Systemic Disease Features

Bursitis and tenosynovitis are associated with RA. Median nerve compression, or carpal tunnel syndrome, is also associated because of wrist tenosynovitis. Constitutional features (Matteson, Cohen, & Conn, 1997) such as fatigue and weight loss may occur early and occasionally; inflammation may extend beyond the joints and involve organ systems.

Nodules

Nodules rarely occur in seronegative RA patients but are not uncommon in seropositive patients. They accompany severe disease and reflect the level of disease activity. They develop subcutaneously in pressure areas such as the Achilles tendon, ischial and sacral prominences, finger joints and elbows. They are firm and adherent to underlying tissue. They may regress with therapy as RA improves. Interestingly, the nodules may increase in number with methotrexate therapy, despite improvement of the disease process.

Hematological Features

There is an anemia of RA. Contributors to the anemia (Matteson et al., 1997) include

- Impaired iron utilization
- Reduced erythropoietin levels and ineffective   erythropoiesis with inhibition of production
- Reduced red blood cell life
- Increased phagocytosis of red blood cells by lymph   nodes and synovium

Thrombocytosis is common. It may correlate with the number of joints involved with synovitis. The mechansism is unclear. There are no thrombotic events associated with thrombocytosis.

Eosinophilia occurs and the pathogenesis is unclear. It is associated with high titers of rheumatoid factor (RF) and serum gamma globulins. Pulmonary complications may be associated with eosinophilia.

Lymphadenopathy occurs frequently with active RA. These nodes are often felt in the axillary, inguinal, and epitrochlear areas; they are mobile and nontender. With good control of RA, the lymphadenopathy diminishes.

Felty's Syndrome

This is RA with splenomegaly and leukopenia. It occurs usually in RA patients with longstanding, seropositive, nodular disease with lower extremity ulcerations and hyperpigmentation. A recently recognized variant of Felty's occurs mainly in older adults early in the disease course of RA. They have neutropenia and an increase in large granular lymphocytes in both the blood and bone marrow. Improvement may occur with glucocorticoid therapy and /or immunosuppression (Matteson et al., 1997).

Hepatic Manifestations

Uncontrolled active RA is associated with increased liver enzymes, especially SGOT and alkaline phosphatase. With good RA control, the liver studies return to normal (Matteson et al., 1997). There may be liver involvement with Felty's syndrome in up to 65% of patients. Some patients have portal fibrosis and nodular regenerative hyperplasia and can develop portal hypertension, esophageal varices, and variceal bleeding.

Pulmonary Manifestations

Involvement of lungs is common but very subtle. Pulmonary fibrosis is estimated in about 28% of patients. Autopsy studies indicate 50% incidence of pleural involvement with effusions in inflamed pleura. Persistent effusions can lead to fibrosis. Seropositive RA patients with nodules often have pulmonary nodules in the periphery. They can cavitate and cause effusions and fistulas. Excisional biopsy is often needed to establish the diagnosis and exclude other diseases.

Older individuals extensively exposed to coal dust may develop pneumoconiosis with their RA. Lesions appear suddenly and cause an exacerbation of the RA. They may cavitate. Also, older adults who smoke will have more pulmonary problems.

Cardiac Manifestations

Pericarditis occurs in seropositive patients with nodules. It is usually not symptomatic, but random ECG evaluation and autopsy studies reveal pericardial inflammation in about 50% of patients. It resolves as RA is better controlled. Symptomatic pericarditis responds to NSAIDs and glucocorticoids.

Echocardiograms will reveal about 30% of patients to have valve involvement. However, it is often hemodynamically insignificant, except perhaps in the older client who already has some degree of valvular impairment.

Patients with severe RA and accompanying vasculitis who develop a myocardial infarction are likely to have coronary arteritis as the basis for the occurrence.

Eye Manifestations

Keratoconjunctivitis is the most common ocular problem in RA and affects 10–35% of patients (Gordon & Hastings, 1997). Some patients have only dry eyes; others may have sicca syndrome, which consists of burning, a sensation of a foreign body in the eye, and a mucoid discharge. Episcleritis seems to correlate with RA activity, causing eye redness and pain, with rare changes in visual acuity.

Neurological Manifestations

Nerve compression commonly occurs. Peripheral entrapment seems to correlate with degree and severity of local synovitis (Gordon & Hastings, 1997). The most commonly involved nerves are the median, the ulnar, the posterior branch of the radial nerves, and the posterior tibials. Tinel's sign is elicited by percussing over the carpal tunnel and tarsal tunnel.

Cervical myelopathy can occur with atlantoaxial subluxation. Cord compression can occur and is indicated by a positive Babinski sign, hyperreflexia and weakness. This complication is seen in longstanding, severe, destructive RA.

Vasculitis

In patients with longstanding disease of 10 or more years, a vasculitis can occur. It is seen in small vessels and is associated with many of the clinical manifestations of RA. Nodules begin as small vessel vasculitis. There may be an inherited susceptibility to this complication. Men are affected more than women. Other risk factors for vasculitis in RA include (Harris, 2001a).

- High titer of RF in serum
- Joint erosions
- Subcutaneous nodules
- Number of DMARDs previously taken

Patients with Felty's syndrome are more likely to develop vasculitis. There may also be skin and nailfold infarcts, digital gangrene, and leg ulcers. There may be distal sensory neuropathy which is an ominous sign (Gordon & Hastings, 1997).

DIFFERENTIAL DIAGNOSIS

Differential diagnosis of diseases that must be excluded to make the RA diagnosis clear include the following common disorders (Harris, 2001a):

- *Acute polyarthritis*: This disorder, of particular significance to older males, presents with sudden onset, so that the elderly man can give a date of first signs and symptoms. The syndrome occurs as intense joint pain, diffuse swelling, and limitation, leading to incapacitation in shoulders, elbows, wrists, fingers, hips, knees, ankles and feet. There is pitting edema. It is remitting, symmetrical and seronegative. It is called "benign RA of the aged" (Gordon & Hastings, 1997).
- *Ankylosing spondylitis*: This is differentiated from RA by lack of involvement of small joints, asymmetry of joint involvement, and lumbar spine involvement
- *Calcium pyrophosphate dihydrate deposition disease*: CPDDD is a crystal-induced synovitis differentiated from RA by arthrocentesis and the presence of unicompartmental disease in the wrists.
- *Diffuse connective tissue diseases*: Among these diseases are systemic lupus erythematosis, scleroderma, vasculitis, mixed connective tissue disease-all differentiated from RA because of low titers of RF, and less synovitis.

- *Fibromyalgia*: This disorder is uncommon in older adults, has no synovitis, and has a greater incidence of psychological disturbances compared to elders with RA.
- *Gout*: Gout mimics RA a great deal. RF is found in about 30% of patients with chronic gout.
- *Infectious arthritis*: Viral infections can present with many characteristics of RA. An arthritis often precedes jaundice in viral hepatitis B. Liver tests will differentiate it from RA. Hepatitis C also mimics RA. Therapy for RA can affect the course of this virus, therefore, it is worth considering obtaining a test for hepatitis C in patients with RA prior to therapy.
- *Lyme disease*: This disease closely simulates RA in adults as it has an associated chronic synovitis. Further, the histopathologic evaluation of the synovium does not differ from RA.
- *Osteoarthritis (OA)*: Most elderly people with RA will also have OA. Each resembles the other as the diseases progress. In late stage OA, a reactive synovitis occurs. As RA erodes cartilage, secondary OA changes in bone and cartilage develop. In end stage OA and RA, involved joints appear very similar. The ESR may be elevated in OA but only slightly, and the RF is not found.
- *Polymyalgia rheumatica (PR)*: If there is significant synovitis in PR, RA must be excluded. A history should differentiate shoulder and hip girdle muscle pain from shoulder joint and hip joint pain. Synovial biopsy indicates a mild synovitis in PR compared to RA. It is probably not uncommon for PR and RA to occur together in many older adults, but there is little information in the literature about it.

DIAGNOSIS

The diagnosis is mainly based on clinical judgment and is made based on the American College of Rheumatology (ACR) criteria for classification of rheumatoid arthritis. Any four of the following criteria must be present to make a diagnosis of rheumatoid arthritis (adapted from 1987 American Rheumatism Association revised criteria for the classification of RA):

- Morning stiffness for > one hour
- Arthritis in three or more joints; arthritis of hand joints (wrists, metacarpophalangeal or proximal interphalangeal joints)
- Symmetrical arthritis
- Rheumatoid nodules
- Positive serum rheumatoid factor
- Radiographic changes in hands typical of RA, including erosions or bony decalcification

A history of present illness (HPI) should include (Gordon & Hastings, 1997)

- Chronological account of illness from the onset
- Acute or gradual onset
- Clinical course: duration, frequency, persistence, periodicity
- Location of pain, radiation of pain
- Type of pain: quality, intensity, and character
- Interference by pain with ADLs, IADLs, social life
- Presence or absence of swelling
- Associated symptoms: fatigue, systemic complaints
- Modifying factors: what aggravates it, what relieves it
- Medications used: effect and side effects
- Duration of AM stiffness, how relieved
- Review of joints, periarticular areas, functional indices
- Psychological effects

An assessment should also consider educational, social, and medical histories, including

- Educational background: affects management and outcome
- Financial situation: may affect management and follow through
- Smoking history
- Hormonal therapies
- History of medical problems and surgeries
- Concomitant medical problems

Because RA is a systemic illness, a thorough physical examination is essential, documenting presence and absence of features. It should include the following: See Disease Course and Evaluation for articular and extra-articular assessment of specific regional areas.

- Specific joints: Behavior of specific joints is best recorded utilizing a skeletal figure with common diarthrodial joints that can be checked to indicate activity or deformity in the joint. Check for tenderness, stress pain, synovial effusion, grip strength, and duration of morning stiffness. Check also for subluxation, malalignment, metatarsal prolapse, hammer toes, lax collaterals, and bone on bone crepitus.
- Extra-articular assessment: Note the presence of nodules, digital infarcts, palmar erythema, Raynaud's phenomenon, episcleritis, peripheral neuropathy, and leg ulcers.

USEFUL TOOLS FOR EVALUATION OF THE OLDER ADULT WITH RA (GORDON & HASTINGS, 1997)

- Stanford Health Assessment Questionnaire (HAQ)
- Functional Disability Index (FDI)
- Arthritis Impact Measurement Scales (AIMS)
- Self-report questionnaire for RA: The client checks the ability to do the following using the ranks of "without any difficulty" to "unable to do" (Gordon & Hastings, 1997)
  - Dressing, including tying shoelaces and doing buttons
  - Getting in and out of bed
  - Lifting a full cup to the mouth
  - Walking outdoors on flat ground
  - Washing and drying entire body
  - Bending down to pick up object on the floor
  - Turning faucets on and off
  - Getting in and out of a car
- Functional Capacity Classification (Gordon & Hastings, 1997)
  - Normal function without or despite symptoms
  - Some disability, but adequate for normal activity without special devices or assistance
  - Activities restricted, requiring special devices or personal assistance
  - Totally dependent

Laboratory Results

Patients with RA may have normochromic-normocytic anemia, a mild leukocytosis, or thrombocytosis. The erythrocyte sedimentation rate (ESR) is elevated about 80% of the time (Beers & Berkow, 2000), and rheumatoid factor (RF) is present in about 50% of cases. A high titer of RF, greater than 1:320 is highly specific. Low titers are found in patients with many other diseases and in about 25% of elderly patients without evidence of any disease (C-reactive proteins, CRP).

Early x-ray findings of affected joints may show only soft tissue swelling. Late features include periarticular osteoporosis, narrow joint spaces, and margin erosions (Beers & Berkow, 2000). Synovial fluid aspirate reveals the extent of inflammation by the number of polymorphonuclear neutrophils (PMNs) (Firestein, 2001).

MANAGEMENT

The American College of Rheumatology (www.Medscape/cme/rheum) goals for therapy of RA include

- Symptomatic relief of disease activity
- Improved physical function and reduction of physical disability
- Intervention in slowing or arresting progression of structural damage

Pharmacological Management

DMARDs (disease-modifying antirheumatic drugs) are currently being used as first-line therapy in the early treatment of RA. However, NSAIDs (non-steroidal anti-inflammatory drugs) are still being used in basic therapy for their anti-inflammatory and analgesic effects. There are newer therapies for RA that are just now available that will most likely prevent the kind of joint destruction and deformity that we see today in our older patients.

NSAIDs

Cox-2 inhibitors should be considered over traditional NSAIDs because of their lessened effect on the gastric mucosa and their lack of platelet inhibition. With traditional NSAIDs, gastrointestinal toxicity occurs four times more frequently in older adults (Beers & Berkow, 2000). These drugs will relieve pain, swelling, and inflammation.

Corticosteroids

Low dose prednisone, 5–10 mg/day, can reduce pain and inflammation and has an immunosuppressive effect beneficial in RA. Corticosteroids have a rapid onset of action. When they are instituted, they are tapered and discontinued as soon as is practical. Glucocorticoids may be given as an intra-articular injection with prolonged local relief. Practitioners must always balance the benefits of steroids with the side effects of osteoporosis, hyperglycemia, diminished wound healing, hypertension, elevated lipids, and increased risk of infection. In younger persons there is an effort in medical management to avoid prolonged use of corticosteroids because of these long-term side effects. In older adults our goal is to preserve physical function and maintain independence and the consideration of taking this risk should be made. Low dose prednisone becomes an option because of the benefits of comfort and physical function.

DMARDS

These drugs are started immediately on diagnosis of RA along with prednisone, which is then tapered as the DMARDs become effective. Some of the DMARDs currently used in therapy include

- Methotrexate
- Hydroxychloroquine
- Sulfasalazine
- Gold
- Azathioprine
- D-penacillamine

Methotrexate (MTX) is pretty much the gold standard or standard of care today and may be given alone or supplemented by one of the newer RA medications just recently introduced to the market. It has rapid onset of action and most patients have significant improvement within the first weeks of therapy. The oral MTX given to RA patients is very low dose; however, laboratory tests are done on a routine basis to follow possible side effects. Liver function is monitored every four to eight weeks (Harris, 2001b). CBCs also are monitored for possible bone marrow suppression and GI bleeding. Folic acid is administered 1 mg qd because it reduces nausea and mucous membrane ulcerations that can occur and it also reduces plasma homocysteine levels—an independent risk factor for coronary artery disease (Harris, 2001b). Pulmonary problems are an uncommon effect of low dose MTX and any new cough should be reported to the practitioner. A study of efficacy and tolerance of MTX in older adults concludes that there is no difference in efficacy or toxicity in older adults compared with younger adults (Bologna, Viu, Jorgenson, & Sany, 1996). MTX is contraindicated in older adults with renal insufficiency.

New RA medications

- Etanercept© (Enbrel) used for moderate to severe RA in patients who have not responded to DMARDs. This is a new tumor necrosis factor-a (TNF-a) inhibitor drug that slows progression of disease. There was a review to determine safety and efficacy in patients >65 that demonstrated it to be safe and well tolerated in older adults. The only adverse event of statistical significance was the injection site reaction that occurred more frequently in patients younger than 65 (personal correspondence, George Spencer-Green, 2001). At this time, there is a waiting list to obtain the drug for RA patients. Cost is about $1,000/month.
- Lenflunomide© (Arava) Used with caution in those elders with renal or hepatic insufficiency, it can be used with MTX or instead of it if MTX is ineffective or not tolerated. Cost about $250/month.
- Infliximab© (Remicade) This is a TNF-a inhibitor drug that halts the progression of RA in combination with MTX. Studies indicate that in addition to sustained reduction of signs and symptoms of RA, quality of life ratings are higher with the two-drug combination than with MTX alone (Lipsky et al., 2000). Infliximab is given intravenously in the office setting.

Other RA medications

- Cyclosporine can be used in patients who cannot take MTX and is taken in combination with NSAIDs and hydroxychloroquine.

- Cyclophosphamide, an analogue of nitrogen mustard that has a better therapeutic index and is the alkylating agent of choice for rheumatic diseases requiring this therapy (Steen, 2001).
- Minocycline is another useful drug in RA. It inhibits biosynthesis and activity of metalloproteases that degrade articular cartilage in RA.

On the horizon—stem cell transplants which are the wave of the future according to the Arthritis Foundation (2001a). Rheumatologists in Europe and America are developing guidelines to decide who should be a candidate for treatment. Clearly, it would only be performed on those with severe, life-threatening arthritis who have failed other therapy and who are otherwise in good health. At this time, it is an investigational procedure.

Criteria for Remission of RA

There are six well-tested criteria for determination of clinical remission of RA (Harris, 2001b). Few patients achieve five of the six criteria, indicating that few achieve a true remission. Probably fewer than 25% achieve remission during the first five years of disease management. However, there is a better chance for remission for men and for patients older than 60 years of age. Criteria for complete clinical remission include the following. (Five of the requirements must be fulfilled for at least two consecutive months.)(adapted from Harris, 2001a, p. 994)

- Morning stiffness not to exceed 15 minutes
- No fatigue
- No joint pain
- No joint tenderness or pain on motion
- No soft tissue swelling in joints or tendon sheaths
- Eythrocyte Sedimentation Rate (ESR) less than 30 mm/hr for women, 20 mm/hr for men

Surgical Management

Surgical replacement of joints is usually deferred as long as possible; however, with great disability and loss of function, the benefits of joint replacement may outweigh the risks. Knee and hip replacements can be accomplished in otherwise healthy elders in their eighties and nineties if it means retaining their independence.

Physical Therapy/Occupational Therapy

The goals of physical therapy are relief of pain, reduction of inflammation and preservation of joint integrity and function (Gordon & Hastings, 1997). Major therapeutic interventions are relief of pain, joint protective modalities such as splinting and resting a joint, and exercise therapy. Joint protection is very different for a client with longstanding disease compared to a newly diagnosed patient. Each joint must be assessed and appropriate exercise prescribed. Swollen or unstable arthritis joints are difficult to move and isometric strengthening is useful. Most therapy occurs at home after sessions with the therapist.

Water exercise therapy increases the sense of well-being and is useful to patients. Exercise therapy is important, especially after surgical intervention.

Comfort Care

Rest is recommended during acute flares of RA. It improves the synovitis. At this time, older patients are fatigued, and energy conservation behaviors are effective in developing the ability to intersperse short periods of physical activity with rest. It is detrimental to elderly RA patients. Prolonged rest increases an already age-related loss of aerobic capacity (Beers & Berkow, 2000) as well as muscle strength. This can easily lead to a functional or complete immobility that cannot be reversed.

The pain of RA is due to the inflammatory response caused by rheumatoid factors that combine with IgG and form immune complexes that deposit in the joints. The resulting inflammation leads to proteolytic enzyme production that damages articular cartilage. Synovitis develops from edema and inflammation of the synovial membrane and joint capsule. Thick layers of granulation tissue, called pannus, develops. Pannus invades the cartilage and eventually destroys the joint capsule and bone. Fibrous tissue and scar formation now occlude the joint space, causing bone deterioration and malalignment. At this point obvious deformity and abnormal joint articulation are visible. Finally, fibrous tissue calcifies, at which time there is total immobility.

The relief of pain is a major goal of RA therapy. Pain can be the factor that limits the effectiveness of physical therapy and occupational therapy. Further, it is a major cause of depression. Pain relief can include use of heat or cold, although this relief is usually transient. Local injections of corticosteroids allow moderate to long-term relief for superficial joints, bursae, and tendons. NSAIDs, especially COX-2 inhibitors are playing a major role in pain control even in patients with long-standing RA. See chapter 3, pain management.

NURSING MANAGEMENT

The geriatric nurse has an important role to play in the management of the older adult with RA. The nurse's support can positively affect self-care and ultimately improve quality of life. Some nursing diagnoses that are appropriate for the older adult with RA include (Luggen & Luggen, 1998):

- Alteration in role performance related to crippling effects of RA
- Impaired physical mobility related to pain and joint deformity
- Pain related to joint inflammation
- Ineffective coping related to depression of chronic illness

Interventions and Outcomes

Alteration in role performance related to crippling effects of RA

Expected outcome: The patient will learn to function in usual roles as much as possible.

Nursing Interventions

- Provide emotional support and encourage expression of fears about dependency, disability, body image, and self-esteem. Support efforts to maintain roles.
- Encourage patients to wear street clothes rather than nightwear, whether they are living at home or in a long-term care setting.

Wearing makeup or nail polish may assist in improving the female's self-concept (Ignatavicius, 2001).

- Churches, social groups, and family can help provide conversation and companionship to avoid the isolation, which can occur with disability. Refer to the Arthritis Foundation, with local chapters in many communities, for many self-help groups and activities and lectures that may assist disabled elders to become more involved in society and more productive.

Impaired physical mobility related to pain and joint deformity

Expected outcome: The patient will achieve the highest level of mobility possible given the limitations of the disease process.

Nursing Interventions:

- Monitor morning stiffness duration. Encourage warm baths morning or evening to decrease stiffness and analgesic needs.
- Give support to ensure the patient's adherence to a prescribed physical therapy program.
- Provide access to assistance devices such as zipper pulls, wide-grip eating utensils, easy-to-open cartons and beverages. There are many tools available to assist in self-care, for example, a long-handled shoe horn, or shoes and clothes with velcro closures. Many are available through the Arthritis Foundation (2001b). Those who assist the elder with self-care are should be aware that utensils may be problematic. Styrofoam and paper cups collapse and bend. A hard plastic cup with a thick handle may be more comfortable.

Pain related to joint inflammation

Expected outcome: The patient will report diminished pain.

Nursing Interventions

- administer analgesics as prescribed. Assess effectiveness utilizing a formal pain tool (see chapter 8).
- Monitor for adverse reaction to medications.

- Try pain-relief measures such as heat, rest, or warm soaks
- Paraffin dips are used by many RA patients in the home setting to ease the pain and stiffness that occur in the morning hours.
- The use of music for the purpose of relaxation and other complementary therapies should be considered (Ignatavicius, 2001).

Ineffective coping related to depression of chronic illness

Expected outcome: The patient will identify two new coping mechanisms.

Nursing Interventions

- Investigate coping strategies that have worked well for the patient in the past.
- Give positive reinforcement for the patient's coping skills.
- encourage verbalization of feelings.
- administer antidepressant medications and monitor their effect and adverse reactions.
- Because RA is a progressive disease, worsening over time, assistance from family members, the community, and home health care may be necessary at some point in time to supplement self care. Nurses can refer patients and families to support group, especially the Arthritis Foundation.

Nurses can play a role in improving a sense of well-being in their patients. Ignatavicius (2001) describes a structured nurse-led cognitive-behavioral program for 90 women with RA over an 18–month period. Outcomes indicate that it was positive in assisting them cope with RA and that these changes were maintained over a 3–month followup period.

Nutrition

Many patients follow special diets to self-treat their arthritis. Practitioners will not know this unless they ask. Books and articles abound with ideas for self-treatment. Some treatments prohibit entire food groups (Gordon & Hastings, 1997) such as milk products, or meats, or fruits. Fasting may be attempted. Older adults with osteoporosis or on courses of steroid therapy need a sufficient intake of calcium and vitamin D and can ill afford fasting or diets that prohibit food groups.

In one study discussed by Gordon and Hastings (1997), 13 of 50 RA patients had evidence of malnutrition; five severely malnourished. Body measurements and skin thicknesses were significantly lower than controls. Levels of serum albumin, transferrin, zinc, and folic acid were significantly lower in those with RA. These 13 RA patients had more active disease, higher ESRs and higher CRPs. Interestingly, diet did not differ in RA patients and controls.

A nurse or dietician should be able to help plan a healthy diet for the older adult with RA. There is some suggestion in the literature that the addition of antioxidants such as vitamins A, C, and E are useful. Omega 3 fatty acids found in salmon and tuna are said to decrease inflammation and may be considered for the diet (Ignatavicius, 2001).

Older adults are often the victims of schemes to obtain money from those looking for a cure. It is important for there to be educational sessions that emphasize the placebo effect, warn of herbal medicines that can be toxic, teach that there is no scientific evidence that wheat germ and tomato-free diets help RA (Harris, 2001b). Copper bracelets worn by RA patients do not benefit the wearer, but are commonly seen on RA patients.

Obesity is a liability in any adult with arthritis. A healthy weight-control diet will benefit any older adult in many ways, but especially in reducing the load on weight-bearing joints.

CONCLUSION

Rheumatoid arthritis is thought of by most practitioners as a disease of middle-age adults. Little thought is given to the progressive nature and debilitation that occur as these patients reach old age. There is very little information in the literature specifically looking at RA in older adults. However, there are contradictory research reports that suggest that there is a clinical subset of RA in older adults. Clearly, there is a need for research in care of older adults with rheumatoid arthritis, including descriptive research of the most basic nature if we are to make significant improvement in our care of this population.

REFERENCES

Arthritis Foundation, (2001a). Stem-cell transplants: A cure for arthritis? *www.arthritis.org/news_stemupdate.asp*

Arthritis Foundation. (2001b). Rheumatoid arthritis. www.arthritis.org/Answers/DiseaseCenter/ra.asp

Beers, M. H., & Berkow, R. (Eds.). (2000). *The Merck manual of geriatrics*, (3rd ed.). Whitehouse Station, NJ: Merck Research Laboratories.

Bologna, C., Viu, P., Jorgenson, C., & Sany, J. (1996). Effect of age on the efficacy and tolerance of methotrexate in rheumatoid arthritis. *British Journal Rheumatol 35(5)*, 453–457.

Firestein, G. S. (2001). Etiology and pathogenesis of rheumatoid arthritis. In S. Ruddy, E. D. Harris, Jr., & C. B. Sledge (Eds.) *Kelley's textbook of rheumatology* (6th ed., vol. 2, pp. 921–966). Saunders: Philadelphia.

Gordon, D. A. & Hastings, D. E. (1997). Clinical features of rheumatoid arthritis: systemic involvement. In J. H. Klippel & P. A. Dieppe (Eds.), *Practical rheumatology* (pp. 169-182). St. Louis: Mosby.

Harris, E. D. (2001a). Clinical features of rheumatoid arthritis. In S. Ruddy, E. D. Harris, Jr. & C. B. Sledge (Eds.) *Kelley's textbook of rheumatology* (6th ed., vol. 2, pp. 967–1000). Saunders: Philadelphia.

Harris, E. D. (2001b). Treatment of rheumatoid arthritis. In S. Ruddy, E. D. Harris, Jr. & C. B. Sledge (Eds.), *Kelley's textbook of rheumatology* (6th ed. vol. 2, pp. 1001–1022). Saunders: Philadelphia.

Ignatavicius, D. D. (2001). Rheumatoid arthritis and the older adult. *Geriatric Nursing, 22(3)*, 139-142.

Kaipiainen-Seppanen, O., Aho, K., Isomaki, H., & Laakso, M. (1996). Shift in the incidence of rheumatoid arthritis toward elderly patients in Finland during 1975–1990. *Clinical and Experimental Rheumatology 14(5)*, 537–42.

Lipsky, P. E. et al. (2000). Infliximab and methotrexate in the treatment of rheumatoid arthritis. *NEJM 343(22)*, 1594–1602.

Luggen, A. S., & Luggen, M. E.(1998). Arthritis and musculoskeletal/immunological disorders: Osteoporosis, mobility issues, pain and comfort. In A. S. Luggen, S. S. Travis & S. Meiner (Eds.), *NGNA core curriculum for gerontological advanced practice nurses* (pp. 435–446). Thousand Oaks, CA: Sage.

Matteson, E. L., Cohen, M. D., & Conn, D. L. (1997). Evaluation and management of early and established rheumatoid arthritis. In J. H. Klippel & P. A. Dieppe (Eds.) *Practical rheumatology*. (pp. 191–198). St. Louis: Mosby.

Mavragani, C. P. & Moutsopoulos, H. M. (1999). Rheumatoid arthritis in the elderly. *Experimental Gerontology 34(3)*, 463–471.

Stein, C. M. (2001). Immunoregulatory drugs. In S. Ruddy, E. D. Harris, Jr., & C. B. Sledge (Eds.), *Kelley's testbook of rheumatology*, (6th ed., vol. 2, pp. 879-898). Saunders: Philadelphia.

4

Gouty Arthritis

Sue E. Meiner

Gouty arthritis (gout) is a crystal-related arthropathy seen in older adults and manifested by severe joint inflammation caused by urate crystal deposits. It is a metabolic disease characterized by recurrent episodes of acute distal mono- or oligo-arthritis, and it is thought to be associated with an inborn error of uric acid secretion or metabolism. The first signs of gout are often reported as a recurrent, sudden onset of pain early in the morning that diminishes within a week. The specific complaints include warmth at the site with swelling, cutaneous erythema, and severe pain. The initial episode usually occurs in the metatarsophalangeal (MTP) joint, or the big toe in 50% of patients. While similar symptoms are experienced by the other 50% of sufferers, the MTP joint is not the initial target for them. Regardless of the joint that is involved initially, fever, chills, and malaise accompany each episode of gout. Over time the attacks become more frequent and usually involve a joint such as the knee, wrist or ankle, elbow bursa, heel or fingers (Gallagher & Sommer, 1999). This disease has four phases that are significant to understand as treatment is planned for the older adult.

EPIDEMIOLOGY

The incidence of gouty arthritis has increased significantly over the past 30 years. According to Brewer and Angel (2000), an estimated 500,000 people in the United States have gout. It is the most common form of inflammatory joint disease in men over the age of 40 (Yoshikawa, Cobbs, & Brummel-Smith, 1998). Gout occurs less frequently in women and then exclusively after menopause. Women who develop gout later in life have twice the prevalence of hypertension, renal insufficiency, and are usually taking diuretics (Puig, et al., 1991). These factors are believed to precipitate the initial acute episode of gout.

Gout is classified as primary—inherited deficit of purine metabolism leading to increased or decreased renal excretion. Eighty percent of cases (95% male) have primary gout, which usually begins in the fourth or fifth decade of life.

Secondary gout, or acquired gout, occurs following hematopoietic or renal disorders. Multiple myeloma, polycythemia vera, and leukemia have increased cell turnover with increased uric acid production. Gout may also develop after chemotherapy or after radiation therapy with massive destruction of cells. Renal disorders that have a diminished excretion of uric acid may also cause secondary gout.

Another mechanism for gout is alcohol intoxication, starvation, and increased serum uric acid levels from inhibition of renal excretion due to lactic acidosis and ketosis. Further, aspirin, thiazides, some diuretics, and tuberculosis medication may also lead to secondary gout.

PATHOPHYSIOLOGY

Although the actual cause of gout is unknown, elevated levels of uric acid in blood and urine are present in association with other signs and symptoms. Uric acid is a metabolite of the purines, which are adenine and guanine. Normally, about two thirds of the uric acid produced each day is excreted through the kidneys. One third is excreted through the gastrointestinal tract.

The kidneys handle uric acid through mechanisms of filtration, reabsorption, and secretion. This complex mechanism begins with uric acid being freely filtered by the glomerulus. This is followed by complete uric acid reabsorption in the proximal tubules. A final secretory action occurs at the distal tubule when the uric acid is returned to the tubular fluid. This final step is responsible for the concentration of uric acid in urine. When the kidneys are damaged, less uric acid is eliminated by the renal system and more is eliminated by the gastrointestinal system (Bancroft & Pigg, 1998).

Asymptomatic hyperuricemia is usually found on routine laboratory examinations (high serum uric acid levels >8 mg/dL in men and > 7 mg/dL in women) or when another problem is presented to the primary care provider. Most persons with hyperuricemia do not develop gout. Therefore, asymptomatic hyperuricemia is a laboratory finding and not a disease (Bancroft & Pigg, 1998). Gouty arthritis symptoms are present with hyperuricemia.

A gout attack occurs when the monosodium urate crystals precipitate within the joint and an inflammatory response is initiated. This usually follows a sudden rise in the serum (blood) urate levels. The urate crystals enter the synovial fluid and are perceived as foreign bodies whereupon the inflammatory cascade is initiated (Bancroft & Pigg, 1998).

Gout progresses through four clinical phases. These begin with asymptomatic hyperuricemia that can progress to acute gouty arthritis. The next progression is from intercritical gout to chronic tophaceous gout. The average time for a person to develop chronic gout is more than 10 years after the first acute episode.

Intercritical gout is that asymptomatic phase that follows recovery from an episode of acute gouty arthritis. During this phase the treatment target is the secondary cause of hyperuricemia. Medications that may have caused an iatrogenic reaction must be identified and either changed or eliminated from the treatment plan whenever possible. Some medications that can precipitate drug interactions are cimetidine (Tagament), erythromycin, tolbutamine (Orinase), ampicillin, and amoxicillin (Smeltzer & Bare, 1996).

Chronic tophaceous gout is identified on radiographs as chalky deposits of sodium urate at a variety of joint sites. Hands and feet are the most affected sites. When joints are affected, tophaceous gout can result in destructive arthropathy and chronic secondary osteoarthritis.

Although gout is a chronic condition, it can be controlled with lifestyle changes and medications in the overwhelming majority of cases. Joint changes that occur with subsequent attacks are permanent.

CLINICAL FEATURES IN OLDER ADULTS

Several factors have been identified as predisposing an older person to gout. These risk factors include lifestyle elements of obesity, high purine diet,[1] and habitual alcohol ingestion. Hypertension and hypertriglyceridemia have been associated with gout. An iatrogenic reaction to the use of diuretics, especially thiazides that block the excretion of urates by the kidneys has also been identified as a risk factor. When hypertension is being treated with a thiazide diuretic and gout symptoms arise, another choice of diuretic must be used unless another form of antihypertensive medication is selected. Another area less identified pertains to trauma in the immediate past medical history of patients with symptoms of gout (Lueckenotte, 2000). The association of trauma, body stressors, and changes in metabolism that can occur are suspect in uric acid changes. In 90% of older adults diagnosed with gout, the high level of uric acid in the blood (hyperuricemia) is primarily due to underexcretion instead of overproduction of uric acid. As with younger adults, urate crystals can deposit in the joints, kidney, or in subcutaneous tissue (tophi). The reasons for this change in physiology can be found in genetic predisposition to a defect of purine metabolism. A family history of gout usually confirms the genetic predisposition (Bancroft & Pigg, 1998).

DIAGNOSIS

During the initial contact with the patient, diagnostic tests and procedures should follow the health and family history and physical examination. The type of gouty arthritis and the causative factors will determine the treatment plan. Medications will be prescribed to relieve inflammation, to control pain, to decrease levels of uric acid by enhancing renal secretion, and to decrease synthesis of uric acid.

---

[1]*Purine*—any one of a large group of nitrogenous compounds that are produced as end products in the digestion of certain proteins in the diet, but some are synthesized in the body. Purines are also present in many medications and other substances, including caffeine, theophylline, and various diuretics, muscle relaxants, and myocardial stimulants. Hyperuricemia may develop in some people as a result of an inability to metabolized and excrete purines.

The following information can assist in making a definitive diagnosis.

Presenting symptoms frequently start at night and may be precipitated by excessive exercise, certain medications, foods, alcohol, or dieting. The patient observes an abrupt onset of pain with redness and swelling. Some patients report that the presence of a bed sheet over the affected joint can produce extreme pain.

A definitive diagnosis of gout can be made only when monosodium urate crystals are in the synovial fluid or in tissue sections of tophaceous deposits. Synovial fluid analysis is useful in excluding other conditions such as septic arthritis, pseudogout (caused by a different pathology), and rheumatoid arthritis.

Once the basic diagnosis is made, it is necessary to identify the cause prior to planning for treatment. Determining if gout is related to overproduction or underexcretion of uric acid is vital. Collecting a 24–hour urine specimen after the patient has begun a purine-free diet will assist in identification of the cause. Urate urine values above the normal range of 264 to 588 mg/day indicate an overproduction of uric acid. Normal serum urate concentration is 5.0 to 5.7 mg/dl in men and 3.7 to 5.0 mg/dl in women. If an overproduction is not identified, then underexcretion is considered to be the cause and treatment will be planned accordingly.

Differential Diagnosis

Rheumatoid arthritis can be mistaken for gout when subcutaneous tophi are evident. Other differentials include cellulitis, hemarthrosis, traumatic joint injury, septic arthritis, or pseudogout (Kennedy-Malone, Fletcher, & Plank, 2000). Pseudogout occurs mainly in knees, wrists or shoulder joints. It is a disorder caused by calcium pyrophosphate dihydrate crystals (CPPD) and presents as an acute oligoarthritis (Yoshikawa et al., 1998). It is associated with metabolic stress such as the postoperative period, trauma, or severe illness. The practitioner may see high fever and increased white blood cell count. It may continue as a chronic polyarthritis resembling RA. The diagnosis is made by the presence of chondrocalcinosis on x-ray or positional birefringent crystals in synovial fluid. Therapy for pseudogout includes NSAIDs, local corticosteroid injections, or colchicine (Yoshikawa et al., 1998).

MANAGEMENT

The goal of treatment is to provide pain relief, prevent further acute episodes, and prevent destructive arthropathy and formation of kidney stones (Gallagher & Sommer, 1999). The prognosis is good. When illness management is initiated promptly, the attack will subside.

Pain Control Measures

Nonsteroidal anti-inflammatory drugs (NSAIDs) are the first-line treatment to reduce the acute painful attack of gout. The most common medications in the NSAID group are indomethacin (Indocin®), ibuprofen (Motrin®), naproxen (Naprosyn®), sulindac (Clinoril®), piroxicam (Feldene®), and ketoprofen (Orudis®). The medication that is prescribed should be taken at maximum dosage until the acute attack has been relieved for at least 24 hours. After the first 24 hours, the dosage can be reduced rapidly for the next two to three days. A complete resolution can be seen in nearly 90% of patients within five to eight days after NSAID medications for pain and anti-inflammation are given at the onset of the attack (Harris, Siegel, & Alloway, 1999). Many patients get relief from an injection of corticosteroids in the affected area.

Pharmacotherapeutics

The primary care provider commonly prescribes colchicine for an attack of gout. Although this treatment can be effective in reducing or eliminating the symptoms of gout, elderly patients commonly have gastrointestinal side effects, even at therapeutic dosages. These side effects include abdominal pain, nausea and vomiting, and/or diarrhea. Older patients with liver or kidney disease are rarely candidates for colchicine therapy. Further, this drug has hematologic and CNS side effects (Yoshikawa et al., 1998). Caution is needed when the patient's medications include cimetidine (Tagamet®), erythromycin, or tolbutamine (Orinase®) due to drug interactions (Gershman & McCullough, 1998).

Another medication frequently prescribed is probenecid to decrease the level of uric acid by enhancing renal secretion. Careful monitoring of the renal status of the older adult is necessary. Probenecid side effects include stomach upset and allergic dermatitis. The patient needs to be advised to report any skin rashes that occur after beginning probenecid therapy.

In some instances, Allopurinol decreases the synthesis of uric acid and is most often used for long-term therapy for gout. It prevents gouty attacks and tophaceous deposits (Yoshikawa et al., 1998). It is most often prescribed for patients who have an overproduction of urate instead of an exogenous cause such as a diet high in purines. Minor side effects can be skin rash, diarrhea, headache and stomach upset. Serious side effects include alopecia, fever, lymphadenopathy, bone marrow suppression, and liver and/or kidney toxicity. In some instances, Allopurinol can induce a gout attack and colchicine is usually prescribed concomitantly. Dosages should be adjusted to keep the uric acid level less than 6 mg/dl and reduced in renal insufficiency. Caution is needed when the patient's other medications include either ampicillin or amoxicillin due to drug-drug interactions (Gershman & McCullough, 1998). Older adults are generally started on a low dose (1/3 of the usual adult dose). A thorough medication list of prescribed and over-the-counter (OTC) drugs currently being taken is necessary prior to planning pharmacotherapeutic interventions for a specific patient. See Table 4.1 for a list of medications associated with the treatment of gouty arthritis.

TABLE 4.1 List of Medications that may be Prescribed for Treatment of Gouty Arthritis

Acetohexamide	Dicumarol	Phenolsulfonphthalein
ACTH	Diflunisal	Phenylbutazone
Ascorbic acid	Estrogens	Probenecid
Azauridine	Glucocorticoids	Radiographic contrast agents
Benzbromarone	Glyceryl guaiacolate	Salicylates (>2g/2d)
Calcitonin	Glycopyrrolate	Sulfinpyrazone
Chlorprothixene	Halfenate	Tetracycline that is outdated
Citrate	Meclofenamate	Zoxazolamine

Note: From "Medications with Uricosuric Activity," by R. L. Wortmann, 2000, *Harrison's Principles of Internal Medicine*, 14th ed. (CD-ROM). New York: McGraw-Hill.

Patient Education

Commonly a patient does not consider the role that diet may play in precipitating an initial attack. The nurse needs to instruct the patient/family on the important role that diet and consumption of alcohol play in stimulating episodes of gout. Discussions on lifestyle modifications are needed to assist in the prevention of an immediate relapse (Lueckenotte, 2000).

Referral to a therapeutic dietitian is strongly recommended to assist the patient in meal planning to reduce or eliminate purine-rich foods (Smeltzer & Bare, 1996). Although diet and lifestyle modifications are the target of treatment, following a rigid restriction of purines is rarely helpful in preventing recurrences. However, instructions in avoidance of foods high in purines, but not a total restriction, may be useful in some instances. Foods that are high in purines increase uric acid in the blood and can stimulate the progression of gout. Foods that are contraindicated because of a high concentration of purines are sardines (in oil), liver, kidneys, anchovies, herring, mussels, and codfish. Other foods that have a moderate amount of purines include scallops, trout, bacon, salmon, veal, venison, turkey, asparagus, beef, bouillon, chicken, crab, duck, ham, kidney beans, lentils, lima beans, mushrooms, lobster, oysters, pork, shrimp, peas, and spinach. Foods that have a low amount of purine includes carbonated beverages, milk, coffee, cheese, eggs, nuts, butter, fruits, breads, grains, macaroni and spaghetti, sugar and sweets, tomatoes, and green vegetables (except those mentioned above) especially lettuce (Harris, Siegel, & Alloway, 1999; Luze & Prizy-Tulski, 1997). It may be difficult to eliminate all purines from the diet. Modification and menu plans that use the least amount of foods that are high in purines, or mixing foods with low purine levels are more easily followed. Many practitioners do not prescribe a special diet for gout because it may be adequately controlled with medication (Luze & Prizy-Tulski, 1997).

Unless contraindicated, ample fluid intake is recommended to promote excretion of uric acid through the urinary system. The selection of fluids needs to balance water with fruit juice. Most older adults have a reduced fluid intake, so the encouragement of liquids needs to be ongoing with reinforcement of the need (Black & Matassarin-Jacobs, 1997).

NURSING MANAGEMENT

The basic goals of nursing management are to relieve pain, reduce inflammation of the affected joints, teach about disease management, and provide follow-up evaluations of effectiveness. Averting an attack through recognition of early symptoms and fast action is possible with a successful teaching program.

The following nursing diagnoses are appropriate for the older patient with gouty arthritis:

- Pain, acute or chronic, related to joint inflammation and swelling
- Risk of activity intolerance related to pain
- Impaired physical mobility related to joint deformity and discomfort secondary to disease process
- High risk for injury related to internal physical factor of altered mobility resulting in risk of falls (Luggen & Meiner, 2000; North American Nursing Diagnosis Association, 1992).

Interventions and Outcomes

Pain, acute or chronic, related to joint inflammation and swelling

Expected outcome: The patient will express decrease in discomfort and pain levels following appropriate use of NSAIDs and analgesics.

Nursing Interventions

- Provide patient/family instructions on the careful use of medications with an understanding of side effects that need to be reported to the health care provider
- Review the use of any adaptive equipment recommended
- Instruct patient regarding appropriate follow-up and referrals if given

Risk of activity intolerance related to pain

Expected outcome: The patient will modify activities and patterns of rest to accommodate the limitations due to pain

Nursing Interventions

- Teach the patient to rest the affected area and limit weight bearing if the first MTP joint is involved.
- Provide measures to assist in elevating the involved extremity with the use of hot or cold packs to the area
- Instruct the patient to increase fluid intake up to three liters a day unless contraindicated.

Impaired physical mobility related to joint deformity and discomfort secondary to disease process

Expected outcome: The patient will be able to verbalize understanding of the disease process.

Nursing Interventions

- Teach modifications of lifestyle behaviors that include reduction in high protein and high calorie diets and eliminate alcohol consumption.
- Discuss nutritional information with diet plans at the first possible opportunity.
- Reinforce the nutritional program prepared by a dietitian if weight loss is needed.
- Encourage the patient to espouse health promotion activities to prevent or minimize future episodes.

High risk for injury related to internal physical factor of altered mobility resulting in risk of falls (Luggen & Meiner, 2000; North American Nursing Diagnosis Association, 1992).

Expected outcome: The patient will be free from injury evidenced by absence of falls.

Nursing Interventions:

- Instruct the patient in non-weight bearing exercises to maintain strength and range of motion; physical therapy may be needed for initial instructions.

- Teach the patient to modify activity and rest patterns to avoid fatigue that can lead to loss of balance and falls.
- Encourage the use of assistive devices for balance and walking if the lower extremities are involved in acute or chronic episodes.

SUMMARY AND CONCLUSION

The primary goal of medical and nursing care of the patient with gouty arthritis is to alleviate pain and discomfort while reducing the inflammatory process accompanying the attack. Once that has been achieved, the nurse needs to initiate the patient/family education program to inform and assist the patient/family with lifestyle modifications that are geared to prevent further acute attacks. These modifications include actions to reduce serum and urinary purines. Supportive care will be needed during the initial attack and if further attacks do occur.

The patient with acute or chronic gouty arthritis must incorporate the necessary changes in diet and lifestyle in order to remain as pain free as possible. Drug therapies are an essential component of the nursing care plan and require patient education and reinforcement. While full mobility and the ability to continue self-care is possible with a diagnosis of gouty arthritis, the nursing professional will need to be vigilant for signs of remission and forgetfulness in observing lifestyle changes. Positive reinforcement must be ongoing in order to achieve the mutual goals of the patient with gouty arthritis and the nursing professional.

REFERENCES

Bancroft, D. A., & Pigg, J. S. (1998). Alterations in skeletal function: Rheumatic disorders. In C. M. Porth (Ed.), *Pathophysiology: Concepts of altered health states*. (5th ed.) Philadelphia: Lippincott.

Black, J. M., & Matassarin-Jacobs, E. (1997). *Medical-surgical nursing: Clinical management for continuity of care*. Philadelphia: Saunders.

Brewer, E. J. & Angel, K. C. (2000). *The arthritis sourcebook*, (3rd ed.) Los Angeles: Lowell House.

Gallagher, G. B. & Sommer A. M. (1999). Topics in musculoskeletal care, In S. Molony, C. Waszynski, & C. Lyder (Eds.), *Gerontological nursing, an advanced practice approach*. (pp. 283-309). Stamford, CT: Appleton & Lange.

Gershman, K., & McCullough, D. M. (1998). *The little black book of geriatrics.* Malden, MA: Blackwell Science.

Harris, M. D., Siegel, L. B., Alloway, J. A. (1999). Gout and hyperuricemia. *American Family Physicians* (pp. 1138-1140). Port Townsend, WA: American Academy of Family Physicians.

Kennedy-Malone, L., Fletcher, K. R., & Plank, L. M. (2000). *Management guidelines for gerontological nurse practitioners.* Philadelphia: F. A. Davis.

Lueckenotte, A. G., (Ed.) (2000). *Gerontologic nursing* (2nd ed.), St. Louis: Mosby.

Luggen, A. S., & Meiner, S. E. (2000). *NGNA core curriculum for gerontological nursing.* (2nd ed.). St. Louis: Mosby.

Luze, C. A. & Prizy-Tulski, K. R. (1997). *Nutrition and diet therapy.* Philadelphia: F. A. Davis.

North American Nursing Diagnosis Association. (1992). NANA approved nursing diagnoses. Philadelphia: Author.

Puig, J. G., Michan, A. D., Jimenez, M. L., Perez de Ayala, C., Mateos, F.A., Mapitan, C. D., de Miguel, E., & Gejon, J. (1991). Female gout: Clinical spectrum and uric acid metabolism. *Archives of Internal Medicine, 151,* 726–732.

Smeltzer, S. C., & Bare, B. G. (1996). *Brunner and Suddarth's textbook of medical-surgical nursing* (8th ed.). Philadelphia: Lippincott.

Yoshikawa T. T., Cobbs E. L. & Brunnel-Smith, K. (1998). *Practical ambulatory geriatrics* (2nd ed.). St. Louis: Mosby.

5

Polymyalgia Rheumatica and Giant Cell Arteritis

Laurie Kennedy-Malone

It is quite common for older adults to present to their primary care provider with complaints of musculoskeletal aches and stiffness. For the patient who presents with an abrupt or insidious onset of proximal muscle pain and stiffness coupled with fatigue, fever, and malaise, polymyalgia rheumatica (PMR) must be considered in the differential diagnosis. Giant cell arteritis (GCA), or temporal arteritis as it is also known, is a common primary vasculitis that often occurs in patients with polymyalgia rheumatica. Left untreated, giant cell arteritis can result in irreversible vision loss. Nurses need to familiarize themselves with these two disorders common in older adults and recognize the presenting symptoms as a periarticular condition that requires immediate referral for diagnosis and proper management (Kennedy-Malone & Enevold, 2001).

EPIDEMIOLOGY

Polymyalgia rheumatica and giant cell arteritis are two immunologic conditions that are found predominantely in older adults; it is rare to see a patient with PMR and GCA younger than age 50. The incidence of PMR rises with age. For older adults over age 80, PMR and

GCA occur ten times more frequently than in adults in their fifties (Kennedy-Malone, Fletcher, & Plank, 1999). PMR is more common among Caucasians of European decent than African Americans and is twice as common in women than in men. PMR afflicts one in 1000 persons age 50 and older in the United States. Approximately 4% to 20% of patients who are diagnosed with PMR develop GCA. The annual incidence for giant cell arteritis is 18 cases per 100,000 persons over the age of 50 (Epperly, Moore, & Harrover, 2000). The etiology of PMR remains unknown. However, a relationship between PMR and the presence of HLA-DR4 haplotype suggests a genetic predisposition (Carpenter & Hudacek, 1994). There are no known screening tests for polymyalgia rheumatica or giant cell arteritis.

PATHOLOGY

Polymyalgia rheumatica and giant cell arteritis are inflammatory disorders. PMR and GCA are conditions characterized by an elevation of the erythrocyte sedimentation rate (ESR). Patients with PMR are found to have bursitis, synovitis, and tenosynovitis of the proximal shoulder and hip girdle, causing muscle soreness, limited range of motion due to pain, and subjective weakness. Round cell infiltration and synovial proliferation are found in patients with PMR. Muscle biopsies are negative in patients with PMR. Specific pathologic changes that have been identified in GCA are histiocytic, lymphocytic, and giant cell infiltrations of the wall of arteries. Inflamed arteries cause the specific symptoms that patients manifest. For instance, patients with an inflamed maxillary artery often present with symptoms of jaw claudication. When arteries supplying the structure of the eye are affected, rapid visual manifestations (flashes, colors, distortions) are the result of the local vasculitis. (Epperly, Moore & Harrover, 2000; Goroll & Mulley, 2000).

CLINICAL FEATURES IN OLDER ADULTS

Polymyalgia Rheumatica

When patients present with polymyalgia rheumatica for the first time they often report that prior to the recent onset of musculoskeletal pain, fatigue, malaise and other associated symptoms, their health status has been generally good. Polymyalgia rheumatica is a systemic disorder. Initially patients complain of muscle aches in the shoulder, pelvic girdle, upper back, and/or neck area for a month's duration. Attempts at alleviating the pain with over-the-counter analgesics and heat application may provide some relief, however in most cases the pain becomes severe. Patients may report unilateral bursitis in the shoulder initially but generally the pain progresses symmetrically (Epperly, Moore, & Harrover, 2000).

As the pain progresses, patients may report inability to get out of bed in the morning without extreme difficulty. The early morning stiffness reported by patients with PMR last longer than 30 minutes. Patients find that they are unable to lift their arms over their head and have to compensate for personal grooming due to pain in their shoulders. Along with pain that may interfere with sleep or performance of activities of daily living, patients often relate feeling of fatigue, malaise, and depression. Underlying fear and anxiety are often manifested due to a suspicion of an unidentified cancer (Carpenter & Hudacek, 1994).

Fever is a common presentation in patients with PMR. They may report episodes of night sweating. When patients are describing their onset of PMR, they need to be questioned also about anorexia and weight loss associated with the disease process (Epperly, Moore & Harrover, 2000; Kennedy-Malone et al., 1999).

When examining a patient you suspect may have polymyalgia rheumatica, apply light pressure first when palpating the afflicted area (s) as tenderness may be elicited with even the slightest touch. Although patients report a sense of weakness, a decrease in muscle strength generally is not found in patients with PMR (Mikanowicz & Leslie, 2000). A grade of three or less on the muscle strength grading scale is indicative of disability that may impair one's functional abilities (Lueckenotte, 1997). Patients may report that they have had difficulty grasping small objects. Holding an eating utensil or writing instrument may have become awkward or even painful. Therefore it is important to assess for signs of carpal tunnel syndrome. When examining the patient, ask about the presence of numbness or tingling sensation of the thumb, index, and middle finger (Carpenter & Hudacek, 1994). Often patients with PMR have a normochromic, normocytic anemia; assessing for signs of pallor would be important during the overall examination (Epperly, Moore, & Harrover, 2000).

Giant Cell Arteritis

It is important to evaluate all patients with suspected PMR for signs and symptoms of giant cell arteritis. Patients need to be questioned for any incidences of recent visual disturbances; temporal or occipital headaches; jaw, tongue, or ear pain (Madan, Drehmer, & Donnelly, 2000). The headache is atypical for the patient; the localization of the pain is different than what the patient has experienced in the past (Epperly, Moore, & Harrover, 2000). In reviewing the patient's recent history, assess for any recent sore throats, hoarseness, or cough. Patients may report that they have noticed scalp tenderness while grooming their hair (Mikanowicz & Leslie, 2000). Assess if the patient is having any pain while chewing and if this is a new experience (Kennedy-Malone & Enevold, 2001).

For patients complaining of visual changes, ask who performs their professional eye examination, what was the date of their last examination, and if they followed through on the recommendations for visual care (Kennedy-Malone & Enevold, 2001). It will be essential to relate this information to the primary care provider if referral to an ophthalmologist becomes necessary. Palpation of the temporal and/or occipital arteries may elicit tenderness; note if there is erythema or swelling at the site of these arteries.

Patients with giant cell arteritis are also at risk for developing an aortic aneurysm as a result of the vasculitis that may result in aortic arch syndrome (Goroll & Mulley, 2000). For those patients with additional known risk factors for abdominal aortic aneurysms (hypertension, and peripheral vascular disease), a thorough abdominal examination to evaluate the presence of bruits is warranted (Kennedy-Malone, et al., 1999).

DIAGNOSIS

The determination of the clinical diagnosis of PMR and GCA begin with positive findings on the history and physical (see Figure 5.1). It will be important for the patient's primary care provider to differentiate PMR from a number of other conditions with similar clinical

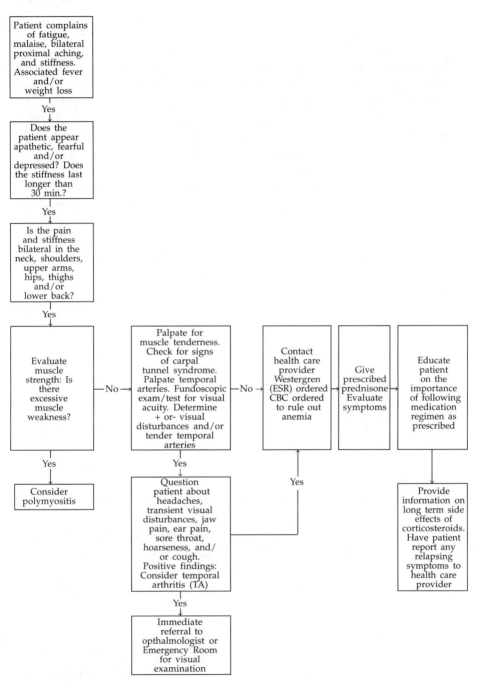

FIGURE 5.1 Polymyalgia rheumatica

Adapted with permission from "Polymyalgia rheumatica," by L. Kennedy-Malone, K. Fletcher, and L. Plank. 1999, *Management Guidelines for Gerontological Nurse Practitioners*, p. 334. Philadelphia: F. A. Davis.

presentation such as elderly onset rheumatoid arthritis (EORA), polymyositis, fibromyalgia, hypothyroidism, and certain cancers. Differential diagnosis of giant cell arteritis includes trigeminal neuralgia, dental conditions, and retinal vascular accident (Dwoltzky, Sonnenblick, & Nesher, 1997; Epperly, Moore, & Harrover, 2000). The clinical hallmark for polymyalgia rheumatica is an elevated Westergren erythrocyte sedimentation rate (ESR). It is common to see reports of ESR greater than 50mm/hr and a reading may exceed 100 mm/hr. In patients with giant cell arteritis, the ESR is often above 100 mm/hr. Supporting laboratory tests for patients with suspected PMR would be a CBC with indices as over half the patients with PMR have a normocytic normochromic anemia. There would be little value in ordering other immunologic studies such as rheumatoid factor and antinuclear antibodies (ANA) because these tests often show elevated levels in asymptomatic older adults (Kennedy-Malone et al.). It is important to note that patients with PMR and GCA may initially have normal ESRs, yet are symptomatic with a milder form of the disease (Brigden, 1999; Epperly, Moore, & Harrover, 2000; Goroll & Mulley, 2000).

In 1990, the American College of Rheumatology identified criteria for the classification of giant cell (temporal) arteritis. A patient with at least three of the five criteria listed, is said to have giant cell arteritis (Hunder, et al., 1990).

1. Age at disease of onset ≥ 50 years
   Development of symptoms or findings beginning at age 50 or older
2. New headache
   New onset of or new type of pain in the head
3. Temporal artery abnormality
   Temporal artery tenderness to palpation or decreased pulsation, unrelated to arteriosclerosis of cervical arteries
4. Elevated erythrocyte sedimentation rate
   Erythrocyte sedimentation rate ≥ 50 mm/hour by the Westergren method
5. Abnormal artery biopsy
   Biopsy specimen with artery showing vasculitis characterized by a predominance of mononuclear cell infiltration or granulomatous inflammation, usually with multinucleated giant cells

Patients experiencing visual disturbances, jaw or mouth pain, and onset of a new headache should be referred to an ophthalmologist for evaluation of giant cell arteritis and possible temporal biopsy. Arterial biopsy is considered the gold standard for diagnosing patients with giant cell arteritis (Epperly, Moore, & Harrover, 2000). Less invasive procedures such as color duplex ultrasonography are being considered as alternative or complementary to the temporal biopsy (Goroll & Mulley, 2000).

MANAGEMENT

Oral corticosteroids continue to be the standard choice of treatment for PMR and GCA in older adults. Almost immediately after a patient is placed on corticosteroids, prompt symptomatic relief of the muscle aches and pain is achieved (Apgar, 1999; Goroll & Mulley, 2000). If a patient does not respond to the corticosteroids, the diagnosis of PMR may need to be reconsidered. The ideal starting dose for PMR and GCA continues to be debated by some authorities; however, if a patient is diagnosed with GCA, the starting dose of corticosteroids generally is higher than if the patient is considered only to have PMR (Hayreh, 2000). Nonsteroidal anti-inflammatory drugs (NSAID) are not recommended for the initial treatment of PMR or GCA (Goroll & Mulley, 2000).

Although there are no preventive measures for PMR or GCA, nurses can educate patients with a prior history of these disorders to report any prevailing signs and symptoms of these inflammatory conditions. Relapses after completion of steroid therapy are common (Kennedy-Malone & Enevold, 2001). Despite the almost rapid cessation of symptoms following introduction of steroid therapy, patients must be instructed on the importance of completing the medication regimen as prescribed. Once the symptoms of PMR and/or GCA are alleviated, the patient's primary care provider will begin to taper the corticosteroid dosage. Included in the education for patients with PMR and GCA must be information on the long-term complications of corticosteroid therapy such as osteoporosis, fractures and infection (Epperly, Moore, & Harrover, 2000). The long-term use of corticosteroid therapy is associated with the risk of developing diabetes, peptic ulcers, cataracts, weight gain and depression (Leslie, 2000).

NURSING MANAGEMENT

The following nursing diagnoses are appropriate for the nursing management of the older adult with PMR and GCA:

- Pain, chronic pain related to chronic disease
- Self-care deficit of ADLs and IADLs
- Risk for infection, fracture, hypertension, diabetes mellitus related to long-term steroid therapy
- Body image disturbance/self esteem disturbance related to increased weight gain from long-term steroid therapy and decreased activity

Interventions and Outcomes

Pain, chronic pain related to chronic disease

Expected outcome: The patient will report a satisfactory level of pain and comfort.

Nursing Interventions

- Administer pain medications as ordered and evaluate satisfactory response.
- Assess for side effects of pain medications.

Self-care deficit of ADLs and IADLs

Expected outcome: The patient will maintain present level of ability to carry out ADLs and IADLs.

Nursing Interventions

- Minimize pain level and duration.
- Encourage warm baths for profound morning stiffness until corticosteroids become effective.
- Encourage periods of rest between periods of activity
- Encourage maintaining activity.

- Determine supports for assistance with home and self-care responsibilities.

Risk for Infection, fracture, hypertension, diabetes mellitus related to long-term steroid therapy

Expected outcome: The patient will be aware of early signs of infection and will cooperate with practitioners in regular appointments to follow possible side effects of therapy.

Nursing Interventions

- Teach the patient about signs of infection, and the need for protection from cuts and abrasions.
- Assess the home environment, shoes, and so on, for protection against falls and fractures.
- Assess blood pressure on a regular basis.
- Follow blood sugars on a regular basis.

Body image disturbance/self esteem disturbance related to increased weight gain from long-term steroid therapy and decreased activity

Expected outcome: The patient will understand why there is weight gain, and plan nutrition and activities to limit the weight gain.

Nursing Interventions

- Follow weights.
- Teach nutrition or refer to a dietician.
- Allow time for the patient to discuss feelings about body image.
- Help the patient plan activities within the scope of limitations.

Patients with PMR need to be reassured that this is not a disabling condition and that it is self-limiting, although it may take over a year for the symptoms to resolve completely. It is important to instruct patients on symptoms of GCA and have them report any new changes immediately. PMR and GCA are diseases of the elderly, and thus many older adults already have concomitant chronic medical problems. They need to report any changes in their health status, as the changes may be exacerbations of chronic conditions or a result of the side effects of corticosteroid therapy.

SUMMARY

Polymyalgia rheumatica, although a fairly common clinical disorder in older adults, often goes undetected and thus untreated due to the specific musculoskeletal complaints and related constitutional symptoms that resemble normal aging changes. Nurses caring for older adults, especially those who work with frail elders unable to verbalize pain and discomfort, need to recognize the characteristic signs and symptoms of PMR and refer them for treatment. Patients complaining of any acute visual changes and/or sensation of jaw claudication need immediate referral to an ophthalmologist with suspicion of giant cell arteritis (Kennedy-Malone & Enevold, 2001).

Nurses need to provide reassurance to the patients that given time with the proper medication regimen, the debilitating symptoms of PMR and GCA will resolve. Older adults with these conditions need to balance periods of rest with gradual return to exercise as permitted. Patients need to focus on improving their nutritional status following a period of weight loss and anorexia. By providing information about the progression of PMR and GCA, offering patient education materials, and monitoring the long-term effects of corticosteroids, nurses will assist patients through the recovery process so they can regain an optimal quality of life (Leslie, 2000).

REFERENCES

Apgar, B. (1999). Corticosteroids in patients with polymyalgia rheumatica. *American Family Physician, 60*(3), 954.

Brigden, M. L. (1999). Clinical utility of the erythrocyte sedimentation rate. *American Family Physician, 60*(5), 1443–1450.

Carpenter, D., & Hudacek, S. (1994). Polymyalgia rheumatica: A comprehensive review of this debilitating disease. *Nurse Practitioner, 19*, 50–58.

Dwoltzky, T., Sonnenblick, M., & Nesher, G. (1997). Giant cell arteritis and polymyalgia rheumatica: Clues to early diagnosis. *Geriatrics, 52*(6), 38–40.

Epperly, T. D., Moore, K. E., & Harrover, J. D. (2000). Polymyalgia rheumatica and giant cell arteritis. *American Family Physician, 64*(4), 778–796.

Goroll, A., & Mulley, A. G. (2000). *Primary care medicine: Office evaluation and management of the adult patient* (4th ed.). Philadelphia: Lippincott, Williams & Wilkins.

Hayreh, S. S. (2000). Steroid therapy for visual loss in patients with giant-cell arteritis. *The Lancet, 355*(9215), 1572–1573.

Hunder, G. G., Bloch, D. A. Michel, B. A., Stevens, M., Arend, W. P., Calabrese, L. H. et al. (1990). The American College of Rheumatology 1990 criteria for the classification of giant cell arteritis. *Arthritis and Rheumatism, 33*(8), 1122–1128.

Kennedy-Malone, L., & Enevold, G. (2001). Assessment and management of polymyalgia rheumatica and temporal arteritis in older adults. *Geriatric Nursing, 22*(3), 152–155.

Kennedy-Malone, L., Fletcher, K., & Plank, L. (1999). *Management guidelines for gerontological nurse practitioners.* Philadelphia: F. A. Davis.

Leslie, M. (2000). When the ache is not arthritis. *RN 2000, 63,* 38–40.

Lueckenotte, A. (1997). *Pocket guide to gerontological assessment* (3rd ed.). St. Louis: Mosby.

Madan, R., Drehmer, T. J. & Donnelly, T. J. (2000). Giant cell arteritis: Episodes of syncope and complexity to an unusual presentation. *Geriatrics, 55*(11), 75-6, 79.

Mikanowicz, C. & Leslie, M. (2000). Polymyalgia rheumatica and temporal arteritis. *Nursing Clinics of North America, 35,* 245–252.

6
Cervical and Lumbar Disk Problems

Sue E. Meiner

There are a number of cervical and lumbar problems of older adults. This chapter discusses the most common of these—cervical spondylosis, spinal stenosis, and diffuse idiopathic skeletal hyperostosis. In addition, osteoarthritis, which is discussed in chapter 2, can be a considerable problem of the spine of older adults and may be associated with spondylitis or other spinal problems. Clinical manifestations of osteoporosis (see chapter 7), such as vertebral compression fractures that usually occur in the lumbar and thoracic areas, may be part of the differential diagnosis of back problems in the older adult. Further, lumbosacral strains, the stretching or tearing of muscles, tendons, and ligaments of the lumbosacral area may occur after injury or trauma. Low back pain is a major problem in all adult groups in the United States. Neck and lower back complaints increase with advancing age.

Cervical spondylosis is a narrowing of the cervical canal due to degeneration of the intervertebral disk and formation of bony osteophytes. Spinal stenosis is a narrowing of the spinal canal that causes pressure on the sciatic nerve and spinal cord. This results from bone or soft tissue pressing on the nerve roots or spinal cord. In diffuse idiopathic skeletal hyperostosis (DISH) there is widespread calcification and ossification of spinal ligaments, which may result in a bony ankylosis. It may also occur in peripheral joints with osteophyte spur formation and calcification of ligaments.

EPIDEMIOLOGY OF CERVICAL AND LUMBAR DISK PROBLEMS

Cervical spondylosis is caused by degenerative changes in the cervical spine that occur with aging. More than 80% of adults over the age of 55 have x-ray findings of cervical disk degeneration. Half of those persons with positive findings are symptomatic (Hazzard, Bierman, Blass, Ettinger, Jr., & Halter, 2000). The onset of spinal stenosis is in adults, age 70 and older. Lumbar stenosis is the most common although it can occur at other levels of the spine. The hypertrophy of bone which narrows the spinal canal and neural foramina causes arterial insufficiency (Brown, Bedford & White, 1999). The incidence of diffuse idiopathic skeletal hyperostosis is about 0.5%/year in older adults (Beers & Berkow, 2000). It occurs more commonly in males than in females (2:1). Although the pathogenesis of DISH is unknown, some research suggests a link to increased serum insulin levels and growth hormone. Other information suggests a relationship to vitamin A and retin A derivatives

Ankylosing Spondylitis

Epidemiological findings indicate that genetic and environmental factors play a role in the pathogenesis of ankylosing spondylitis. This disease affects between 2% and 8% of the Caucasian population with positive inherited HLA-B27 antigen findings. However, 90% of all adults diagnosed with ankylosing spondylitis have the HLA-B27 antigen. It is more common in men than in women and when it does occur, the progression of the disease is slower in women than it is in men (Porth, 1998).

Screening for ankylosing spondylitis does not include a routine HLA typing because it is not specifically diagnostic for this disorder. A sedimentation rate (ESR) is performed along with routine blood studies including white and red blood cell analysis. (See Box 6.1 for age-related calculations of ESR.) Mild normocytic and normochromic anemia are frequently identified with this disorder. Radiologic

---

**BOX 6.1 Age-Related Adjustments for the Erythrocyte
Sedimentation Rate (ESR)**

Westergren formula: Women = (age + 10)/2   men = age/2

---

examination is done to identify the appearance of a squaring of the vertebrae instead of the normal concave appearance (Porth, 1998).

Lumbar stenosis is as common as cervical spondylosis in adults 55 years old or older. This diagnosis is a common cause of back and leg pain. Few cases of lumbar stenosis are considered congenital because of the premorbid narrowing of the spinal canal as degenerative changes occur. In most cases, this disorder is attributed to acquired degenerative or arthritic changes of the intervertebral disks (Alvarez & Hardy, 1998).

PATHOPHYSIOLOGY

The pathogenesis of ankylosing spondylitis is not well understood. An immune response is suggested due to the presence of mononuclear cells in acutely involved tissue.

In cervical spondylosis, extensive degeneration of intervertebral bodies occurs with narrowing of disk spaces. Further changes include osteopathic lipping of vertebral bodies and thickening of ligaments. Osteoarthritic changes occur in the posterior vertebral joints. These changes can result in compression of the cervical spinal cord, nerve root, and spinal arteries (Hazzard et al., 2000).

With lumbar stenosis, a narrowing of the lumbar spinal canal occurs. A cartilaginous hypertrophy of the articulations surrounding the canal, intervertebral disk herniations or bulges, spondylolisthesis (subluxation of one vertebra on another), hypertrophy of the ligamentum flavum, and osteophyte formation are other features of lumbar stenosis (Alvarez & Hardy, 1998).

Neurogenic claudication results when the microvasculature of the lumbar nerve roots are compressed and become ischemic. With extension of the spine during standing, degenerated intervertebral disks and thickened ligamenta flava protrude posteriorly into the lumbar canal causing compression on the cauda equina (Alvarez & Hardy, 1998).

CLINICAL FEATURES IN OLDER ADULTS

Cervical spine complaints of localized stiffness and pain of the neck cause the person to seek medical attention. The pain is radicular (involving a spinal nerve root) or nonradicular in nature. In some instances spasticity, hyperreflexia and even myelopathy follow the initial symptoms (Hazzard et al., 2000). When cervical spondylosis with myelopathy is present, a shuffling gait with spasticity can be seen. The person reports that the "legs just gave way." Some adults report that they have become more clumsy and unsteady on their feet (Ebersole & Hess, 1998).

The typical complaint given when ankylosing spondylitis and/or lumbar stenosis are suspected is persistent or intermittent low back pain. The symptoms may be mild in early stages of these disorders. The patient frequently remembers that the back pain has gotten progressively worse over several months to years since it was first noticed. As the discomfort intensified over this period of time, leg fatigue, numbness and weakness were added to the complaint of pain. Once leg pain begins it progresses to the buttocks and thighs and then travels to the feet. This commonly occurs when leg exercises are begun. Symptoms of back and lower back disorders are usually described as burning, cramping, numbness, tingling or dull fatigue in the thighs and legs (Alvarez & Hardy, 1998).

DIAGNOSIS

The health history will contain information about a much earlier beginning to neck and/or back pain that is described as nonspecific. When cervical spondylosis is suspected, the health history will contain symptoms of local and radicular pain with occasional findings of myelopathy and spasticity. In advanced cases weakness, ataxia, and hyperreflexia are present. The history for lumbar stenosis will contain changes that may be insidious or more rapid with the occurrence of leg fatigue, pain, numbness and weakness. Once leg pain begins it is usually bilateral with buttock and thigh pain developing. Rest relieves the pain in most cases. Standing and walking will exacerbate the pain, but certain other exercise activities do not intensify pain. An example of an exercise that can be done without eliciting lower back pain is riding a stationary bicycle.

Physical Examination

The cervical spine physical examination begins with the identification of localized stiffness. Radicular or nonradicular pain needs to be determined by subjective complaints elicited by the exam. Posterior osteophyte formation may cause vascular compression.

Physical examination of patients with potential lumbar stenosis should begin with the back. Curvature of the spine should be noted, as well as degree of flexibility and mobility during the examination. Lumbar spine clinical features include low back pain and stiffness, muscle spasm, and compression causing radicular pain. Recording the presence of leg pain, paresthesias or numbness with extension of the spine is an important finding. Lasegue's sign or the straight leg-raising test will be negative in lumbar stenosis and positive in a herniated lumbar disk. Patrick's sign or lateral rotation of the flexed knee indicates ipsilateral degenerative hip joint disease and not necessarily lumbar stenosis. In severe cases, the lower extremities exhibit generalized weakness with urinary and bowel dysfunction.

The physical examination for suspected ankylosing spondylitis includes taking measurements to determine the fingertip length to the floor in a forward bending, straight knee position, and contralateral flexion of the back. During the forward bending, if pain is present and increases with pressure over the sacroiliac joint, this disorder is not ruled out. Chest expansion at the fourth intercostal space is done to determine if the thoracic spine is also involved. If a normal finding of a 4–5 centimeter increase with inhalation does not occur, further examination of the thoracic spine is indicated.

Diagnostic Tests

During the initial examination, diagnostic tests such as the Tinetti Balance and Gait Evaluation are suggested. This test examines sitting, standing with standing stability, and turning (Tinetti, 1986). The findings from this test will provide a baseline for measurements of movement. This information is important in follow-up visits to assess improvement in gait, balance, and flexibility.

The use of magnetic resonance imaging (MRI) and computed tomographic (CT) scans have provided the techniques to diagnose cervical, thoracic, lumbar, and sacral musculoskeletal diseases. The uses of plain radiographic images are not diagnostic but can demonstrate degenerative changes in the vertebrae or disk spaces. While myelography was used in past decades, it is rarely used today in favor of the MRI and/or CT scanning.

DIFFERENTIAL DIAGNOSES

Among the many differentials for painful disorders involving the cervical spine are subacute combined degenerative joint disease, spinal cord tumor, and early incipient pressure hydrocephalus. Others to consider are osteomyelitis, septic arthritis or discitis, cervical lymphadenitis, thyroiditis, trauma-fractures, meningitis, osteoporosis, and a metastatic tumor (Greenberger, Berntsen, Jones, & Velakaturi, 1998).

Differential diagnosis for lumbar stenosis includes cauda equina compression (syndromes), lumbosacral spinal tumor, lumbar epidural abscesses, compression fractures, and spondylolisthesis. Another area that creates a secondary lumbar stenosis is the reactive bony hypertrophy following a posterior lumbar fusion (Alvarez & Hardy, 1998).

Intermittent claudication from peripheral vascular disease and neurogenic claudication from nerve involvement are difficult to differentiate in older adults with multiple chronic conditions. A neurologist is needed to identify the origin of the symptoms of lower extremity dysfunction (Hazzard et al., 2000).

DISEASE MANAGEMENT

Medical/Surgical Management

Medical management is directed toward pain relief and structural support of the affected vertebrae. Conservative treatments such as cervical or lumbar bracing and bed rest have limited benefits for long-term management. Physical therapy treatments in the form of hot and/or cold applications and selected exercises for the area of spinal involvement are helpful in mild cases. Chapter 8 on assessing and managing pain and Chapter 9 alternative and complementary therapies in arthritis management will provide information related to additional management issues. When symptoms are incapacitating, surgical remedies need serious consideration and in severe cases surgery is the only option to reduce pain and improve stability of the spine (Alvarez and Hardy, 1998). The most common surgical procedures are the anterior cervical dissectomy or the laminectomy. Both include a fusion of the bony structures above and below the point of disk involvement. The overall condition of the patient is of primary concern as the options for treatment are discussed. While older adults can generally tolerate either of these surgeries, comorbid conditions might prohibit either. Major contraindications for surgery would be anticoagulation therapy that is too risky to stop prior to the procedure or severe cardiac or respiratory disease (Tuite et al., 1994).

Surgical risks include reaction from general anesthesia, wound infection, hematoma formation, cerebrospinal fluid leaks, and nerve root damage. In some instances spinal instability results following a decompressive laminectomy. With any spinal surgery, significant pain relief may or may not be the outcome (Alvarez & Hardy, 1998).

NURSING MANAGEMENT

Nursing management should address pain relief and patient safety, with attention to fall prevention. A self-care approach to independent living will need to include mild physical activities to support daily living needs.

The following nursing diagnoses are appropriate for the older patient with arthritis of the spine, ankylosing spondylitis, cervical spondylosis, and lumbar stenosis:

- Pain, acute or chronic, related to arthritis of the spine, intervertebral disk problem
- Impaired physical mobility related to decreased flexibility secondary to disease process
- Potential for fall(s) related to impaired physical mobility

Interventions and Outcomes:

Pain, acute or chronic, related to arthritis of the spine, intervertebral disk problem

Expected outcome: The patient will report minimal discomfort and adequate level of pain control.

Nursing Interventions

- Assess the over-the-counter (OTC) and prescription medicine review, to be included with the health history. Often the older adult with chronic pain takes several remedies that include prescription, OTC, and herbal/food supplement formulations. The importance of obtaining a full and complete list is vital to the understanding of the symptoms. If some symptoms are masked while others are caused by interactions among the various drugs, prescribing additional pain and anti-inflammatory medicines is risky.
- Inform the patient that pain relief can come in forms other than medications. These can be helpful for mild to moderate distress when combined with appropriate anti-inflammatory medications.
- Instruct the patient in nonpharmacologic therapies such as water exercises, heat applications, and anticipatory rest periods during the day.

Impaired physical mobility related to decreased flexibility secondary to disease process

Expected outcome: The patient will be able to verbalize understanding of the disease process

Nursing Interventions

- Expected outcome: non-pharmacologic therapies such as water exercises, heat applications, and anticipatory rest periods during which the patient will continue supportive activities that enhance coping behaviors.

- Patient teaching activities should include a weight reduction program if needed, a smoking cessation program if needed, referral for water exercises, instruction in mild flexibility and balance exercises, and self-concept support.
- Plan for follow-up visits and telephone support.

(Luggen & Meiner, 2000; North American Nursing Diagnosis Association, 1992).

Potential for fall(s) related to impaired physical mobility.

Expected outcome: The patient will be free from injury evidenced by absence of falls.

Nursing Interventions

- Patient safety is a concern due to potential instability in gait and balance. Instruct in the use of mobility aids that are tailored to the patient's needs. Assess and assist in preparing the environment for use of mobility aids.
- A fall prevention program should be instituted whether the patient is in a facility or in a home setting. Safety issues inside and outside of the residence need to be addressed (Ebersole & Hess, 1998; Lueckenotte, 2000).

CONCLUSION

Older adults with degenerative spinal disease of the cervical and lumbar vertebrae can become discouraged readily due to the chronicity of the condition. While treatment is aimed at controlling pain and maintaining mobility by suppressing inflammation, surgery is often the only remedy for spinal instability. Conservative treatments are beneficial to those with mild forms of degeneration but the results are not long lasting. Physical therapy treatments and exercises can prevent injuries due to tripping and falling by increasing the flexibility of the affected vertebrae.

These chronic conditions are a challenge for the patient/family and health care providers. Nursing interventions are important in that they provide the patient with information on the current state of the condition, the expected progression or disease trajectory, and ways to obtain the most comfort while remaining physically active to the maximum possible.

REFERENCES

Alvarez, J. A., & Hardy, R. H. (1998). Lumbar spine stenosis: A common cause of back and leg pain. *American Academy of Family Physicians, 57*(8), 1825-34, 1839-40.

Beers, M. H. & Berkow, R. (Eds.). (2000). *The Merck manual of geriatrics* (3rd ed.). Whitehouse Station, NJ: Merck.

Brown, J. B., Bedford, N. K. & White, S. J. (1999). *Gerontological protocols for nurse practitioners.* Philadelphia: Lippincott.

Ebersole, P., & Hess, P. (1998). *Toward healthy aging: Human needs and nursing responses* (5th ed.). St. Louis: Mosby.

Greenberger, N.J., Berntsen, M.S., Jones, D.K., & Velakaturi, V.N. (1998). *Handbook of differential diagnosis in internal medicine: Medical book of lists* (5th ed.). St. Louis: Mosby.

Hazzard, W. R., Bierman, E. L., Blass, J. P., Ettinger, Jr., W. H., & Halter, J. B. (2000). *Principles of geriatric medicine and gerontology* (4th ed.). New York: McGraw-Hill.

Lueckenotte, A. (2000). *Gerontologic nursing* (2nd ed.). St. Louis: Mosby.

Luggen, A. S., & Meiner, S. E. (2001). *NGNA core curriculum for gerontological nursing* (2nd ed.). St. Louis: Mosby.

North American Nursing Diagnosis Association. (1992). NANDA approved nursing diagnoses. Philadelphia: Author.

Porth, C. M. (1998). *Pathophysiology: Concepts of altered health states* (5th ed.). Philadelphia: Lippincott.

Tinetti, M. E. (1986). Performance oriented assessment of mobility problems in elderly patients. *Journal of the American Geriatric Society 34*, 199.

Tuite, G. F., Stern, J. D., Doran, S. E., Papadopoulos, S. M., McGillicuddy, J. E., Oyedijo, D. I., et al. (1994). Outcome after laminectomy for lumbar spinal stenosis. Part I: Clinical correlations. *Journal of Neurosurgery 81*, 699–706.

7

Osteoporosis

Patricia Mezinskis

Osteoporosis is a degenerative bone condition that results in disability for millions of adults each year. As the older population in the United States continues to grow, osteoporosis will become an even more critical public health challenge. In the past, this disease was considered to be a natural part of aging. However, today health care professionals view osteoporosis as a preventable and treatable disease. Nurses can assist individuals by educating them on the importance of early diagnosis and treatment strategies. Teaching directed toward younger populations can aid in the prevention of this disease and its debilitating consequences.

EPIDEMIOLOGY

Ten million Americans have this disease; 80% are women. Osteoporosis is the predominant metabolic bone disease and many older women do not receive treatment, though they are the most commonly affected population. Another 18 million Americans have low bone mass, which puts them at risk for developing the disease. One out of every two women and one in eight men over age 50 will have a fracture in their lifetime due to osteoporosis (National Resource Center, 2000). Although vertebral fractures occur most frequently, hip fractures have a higher morbidity. Osteoporosis leads to more than 1.5 million fractures each year including (National Resource Center, 2000):

- 300,000 hip fractures
- 700,000 vertebral fractures
- 250,000 wrist fractures
- 300,000 other fractures

Although osteoporosis is considered a disease of older adults, it is also seen in younger populations. It is often referred to as the "silent disease" because it occurs without symptoms. A painful fracture may be the first evidence of the disease. The hospital and nursing home costs associated with osteoporotic fractures is $13.8 billion annually (National Resource Center, 2000).

BONE MASS

An individual's peak bone mass occurs by age 35. It is influenced by many factors, including heredity, adequate calcium, and weight bearing exercise. In the five to seven years following menopause, women lose up to 20% of their bone mass. By age 60 to 70, more than 30% of women have osteoporosis. The incidence increases to 70% of women by age 80 (Taxel, 1998).

RISK FACTORS

Although the exact cause of osteoporosis is unknown, several risk factors have been identified (See table 7.1). According to McClung and Sieber (2000): Osteoporosis occurs most commonly in postmenopausal women, in Caucasian or Asian women, and in women with a low body weight. Additionally, a low calcium intake contributes to bone loss, as does smoking, alcohol consumption, and lack of exercise. A family history of osteoporosis is a risk factor. Some researchers believe that high caffeine intake contributes to this disease

TABLE 7.1 Risk Factors for Osteoporosis

Female
Advanced age
Caucasian or Asian race
Thin body build
Early menopause
Low calcium intake
Smoking
Excessive caffeine/alcohol use
Lack of exercise
Fracture as an adult
Family history of osteoporosis

Adapted from McClung, B., Sieber, A, (2000). Clinical management of patients at risk for or diagnosed with osteoporosis. *Nursing Practice Guide,* Medical Information Services.

(Dannemiller Memorial Education Foundation and Ventiv Health Communications, 2000).

PATHOPHYSIOLOGY

Osteoporosis is defined as a systemic disease characterized by low bone mass and deterioration of the skeletal structures, with a resulting risk of fractures due to porousness of the bones (European Foundation for Osteoporosis and the National Osteoporosis Foundation Consensus Development Statement, 1997). This definition encompasses factors both quantitative and qualitative. The quantity of the osteoporotic bone is actually reduced. The quality of the bone changes when the trabecular struts are thinned. Trabecular bone is the type of thready structure found in spongy or cancellous bone, which provides strength to bone but does not add to its weight. Trabecular bone is found in the vertebrae, pelvic bones, flat bones, and the ends of long bones. Loss of this trabecular architecture leads to a reduction in bone strength and an increased risk of fragility fractures. Though trabecular or cancellous bone is lost first, eventually cortical or compact bone is also lost. Cortical bone is found in the shafts of long bones. Trabecular bone loss occurs about 10 years earlier than loss of cortical bone (Gamble, 1995a).

New bone is formed by osteoblasts, while old bone is destroyed by the action of osteoclasts. This process, known as bone remodeling, occurs approximately every 120 days, as bones cycle through this process of formation and resorption. After peak bone mass is achieved in the mid-thirties, bone resorption, or loss, begins to exceed bone formation. Age-related loss of bone begins in women before men and is accelerated in the first 10 years after menopause. Women may lose 35% of cortical bone and 50% of trabecular bone whereas men may lose 23% of cortical bone and 33% of trabecular bone during their lives (Gamble, 1995a).

Osteoporosis may be the result of decreased osteoblastic activity. The osteoblasts may have a shortened life span or may become less efficient. Another theory is that an increase occurs in osteoclastic, or bone resorption, activity. This theory has gained acceptance in recent years and therapeutic agents have been developed to prevent bone breakdown (Ignatavicius, Workman, & Mishler, 1999).

CLASSIFICATIONS

Osteoporosis is classified as primary or secondary. Primary osteoporosis is further delineated as Type I or Type II. In Type I, rapid bone loss is related to menopausal estrogen loss and is seen in women aged 51–75. Estrogen and testosterone aid in the absorption and use of calcium, needed for maintaining bone. Because estrogen deficiency occurs with menopause and testosterone loss in men occurs more slowly, Type I osteoporosis is seen six times more often in women than in men. Additionally, women are more prone to osteoporosis than men because they have proportionally less bone mass. Type II osteoporosis is evident in both men and women over the age of 70 and occurs with a gradual loss of cortical bone (Van Dyke Lamb, & Cummings, 2000).

Secondary osteoporosis, which is seen in about 15 % of cases, is the result of an underlying etiology. The causes of secondary osteoporosis (Table 7. 2) include a number of medical conditions and long-term use of several medications (Peterson, 2001).

CLINICAL FEATURES/ASSESSMENT

It is important for the nurse to complete a thorough history as well as a physical and psychosocial assessment of the individual to aid in early detection and treatment of osteoporosis. Identifying risk factors is a good beginning. Questions should be asked regarding the risk factors shown in Tables 7.1 and 7.2. Questions should include the woman's age at menopause, amount of calcium intake, history of smoking, and use of caffeine or alcohol. Data should be obtained on the patient's history of fractures and family history of osteoporosis. It is important to ask if the patient has a routine exercise program. The patient should also be questioned about medications taken, such as steroids or antineoplastic agents. Because many illnesses can cause secondary osteoporosis, these areas should also be investigated (see Table 7.2.)

TABLE 7.2 Causes of Secondary Osteoporosis

Alcoholism
Liver disease
Cushing's Disease
Hyperthyroidism
Hyperparathyroidism
Hypogonadism
Malnutrition and malabsorption disorders
Neoplasms
Prolonged immobility
Long term use of certain medications:
    Corticosteroids
    Heparin
    Phenytoin
    Phenobarbital
    Methotrexate

Adapted from Peterson, J. (2001). Osteoporosis overview. *Geriatric Nursing, 22*,(1), 17–21.

STRUCTURAL ASSESSMENT

Frequently, there are no clinical symptoms until a fracture occurs. With a compression fracture of the spine, the vertebra changes from the normal shape into a wedge, with the narrow angle of this wedge on the anterior side of the vertebra. Because of this occurrence, the spine bends forward. It is important to note that vertebral compression fractures often go unreported. When assessing a patient, the vertebral column should be inspected. Individuals should be asked if they have noticed that they are not as tall as they used to be. One study (Hunt, 1996) showed that individuals with the greatest height loss had the lowest bone mass. With osteoporosis, height loss can be quite extensive. A loss of 1.5 inches is typical of the disease, but some individuals lose as much as 4 to 8 inches (Gamble, 1995a). As the disease develops, dorsal kyphosis or the "dowager's hump" may be seen due to numerous vertebral compression fractures.

Because of the deformity of the spine, individuals may have resultant restriction of movement. Both of these problems can lead to respiratory compromise, decreased appetite, abdominal protrusion, and constipation.

Patients may complain of pain, which is generally in the mid-lower thoracic or lumbar area. This chronic pain may be exacerbated with activity such as bending, stooping, or lifting. Palpating patients' vertebrae may also cause them to complain of pain. Following a vertebral compression fracture, acute pain usually lasts 2–3 weeks, though it may last as long as several months (Leslie, 2000).

MOBILITY ISSUES

Patients should be evaluated for any changes in gait and ability to ambulate. Overall frailty can contribute to falls, which can be devastating for the individual with osteoporosis. Hip fractures lead to the most serious outcomes, though they are not as common as vertebral fractures. Approximately 10–20% of persons sustaining a hip fracture die within a year. One quarter of hip fracture patients require long-term nursing home care. Only one third of these patients will regain their former level of independence (National Osteoporosis Foundation, 1998).

PSYCHOSOCIAL ASSESSMENT

A psychosocial assessment is indicated for the patient with osteoporosis. Body image may be affected, especially for the person who has severe kyphosis. Patients may be very conscious of their change in appearance and have trouble finding clothes that fit. Social interactions may have been curtailed due to both the physical limitations that may have occurred but also because of changes in self-image. Someone who has had a very active life may no longer go out or engage in activities that once interested them. Fear of falling or of another fall that might result in fracture may also contribute to isolation and inactivity. A fall risk assessment tool is particularly beneficial for patients living in long-term care institutions.

Depression is not an uncommon result for the person with severe osteoporosis. Inability to continue social contacts can further exacerbate the depression. Patients with osteoporosis who have experienced significant lifestyle changes should be screened for depression and treated as necessary. It is also important to assess for cognitive changes because of the risk of falling in patients with dementia or other cognitive disorders.

DIAGNOSIS

Although x-rays can detect bone loss, at least 30% of bone loss must occur before osteoporosis is apparent with conventional x-rays (Van Dyke Lamb & Cummings, 2000). Today, however, it is possible to predict the risk of fracture by measuring bone mineral density (BMD). The World Health Organization (WHO Study Group, 1994) has established criteria for diagnosing osteoporosis by using standard deviations below the normal mean peak bone mass of young adults. Densitometry is a noninvasive and accurate measurement of BMD based on the way mineralized bone absorbs x-rays. The T-score obtained is the patient's score in standard units based on values from a population of young adults. The WHO has defined osteoporosis in terms of the bone mineral density score, as shown in Table 7.3.

TABLE 7.3 Bone Mineral Density Scores

Diagnosis	T SCORE
Normal	Between +1 and –2 SD
Low bone mass	Between –1 and –2.5 SD
Osteoporosis	Below –2.5 SD
Severe osteoporosis	Below –2.5 SD and one or more fragility fractures

Adapted from WHO Study Group, "Assessment of Fracture Risk and Its Application to Screening for Post-Menopausal Osteoporosis," 1994, *WHO Technical Reports Series*, no. 843. Geneva, Switzerland: World Health Organization.

DIAGNOSTIC TESTS AVAILABLE

Quantitative computed tomography (QCT) has been used to measure bone mineral density of vertebral bone. However, it is costly and delivers a good deal of radiation. Clinicians are using this technique less because of newer methods. Dual energy x-ray absorptiometry (DEXA) can measure bone density of the hip and spine. It is becoming increasingly available and involves less radiation, is economical, and provides high resolution (Maher, Salmond, & Pellino, 1998). DEXA is considered the "gold standard" for the diagnosis of osteoporosis and monitoring of treatment. Peripheral DEXA is now possible for patients unable to move onto the DEXA table. Because of the portability of the equipment, peripheral DEXA is often a good choice for screening (Taxel, 1998). Quantitative ultrasound (QUS) is another diagnostic procedure that provides low cost, portable, radiation-free assessment of BMD using the heel, wrist, or hand (Schoen, 2000).

BMD measurement is recommended for women over 65, postmenopausal women, women with a history of fracture, and those with long-term use of glucocorticoids (such as hydrocortisone, prednisone, or dexamethasone). Also, women who have conditions that can cause secondary osteoporosis (see Table 7.2), should be evaluated (Taxel, 1998).

In July of 1998, Medicare coverage of bone density measurements for the detection of osteoporosis was established after the Medicare

Bone Mass Measurement Act was passed (Dowd & Cavalieri, 1999). This was an important step because the National Osteoporosis Foundation (1998) recommends BMD testing for all women over the age of 65.

Biochemical markers to measure bone formation and resorption have been identified but have not been found to be definitive in the diagnosis of osteoporosis and are not widely used in the clinical setting (Peterson, 2001).

MANAGEMENT

Pharmacologic Treatment

Treatment is aimed at increasing calcium and Vitamin D intake. Other medications have been shown to prevent demineralization of bone and increase bone mineral density. Medications currently being used are shown in Table 7.4.

Calcium

Premenopausal women and postmenopausal women who are taking hormone replacement therapy (HRT) need 1000 mg of calcium each day. For the postmenopausal women not taking HRT, an intake of 1500 mg of calcium is needed. For men and women over age 65, 1500 mg of calcium is recommended (National Osteoporosis Foundation, 1998).

Vitamin D

Fortified milk and egg yolks contain Vitamin D, which is needed for the absorption of calcium. Exposure to sunlight is also a good source of Vitamin D. For people who are institutionalized and unable to get outside, supplementation may be needed. The recommended daily intake of Vitamin D is 400–800 IU/d (Dowd & Cavalieri, 1999; Leslie, 2000).

Sodium Fluoride (investigational drug)

An FDA Advisory Committee has recommended the approval of sodium fluoride which is a slow-release product. Taken with calcium, fluoride has shown promise in increasing bone mass and decreasing the incidence of spinal fractures (Maher et al., 1998).

TABLE 7.4 Pharmacologic Interventions

Drug	Dose	Nursing Implications and Patient Teaching
Calcium	1000–1500 mg. PO	Take in divided doses Take with meals GI distress may occur Monitor for hypercalcemia Take with Vitamin D
Vitamin D (Calcitriol, Ergocalciferol)	400–800 IU/d PO	Side effects include kidney stones Should not be taken if abnormal hepatic or renal function present
Sodium fluoride	25 mg bid PO Investigational drug	Side effects include gastric distress, painful joints Take with food Monitor serum fluoride levels every 3 months BMD studies every 6 months to document progress of bone density Adequate calcium while on this drug
Estrogen Conjugated estrogen (Premarin) Estradiol (Estrace) Estradiol (Estraderm)	0.3–0.625 mg/d PO 0.5mg/d for 3 wk, then off 1 wk 0.05 mg via transdermal patch, applied to abdominal skin twice weekly	Medroxyprogesterone (Provera) 10 mg on days 15–25 may be prescribed to prevent endo-metrial cancer caused by HRT. Instruct client regarding self breast exam, yearly mam-mography, yearly gynecologic exam Report abnormal vaginal bleeding If also on progesterone, instruct on when this is to be taken Encourage client to stop smoking
Bisphosphonates Calcitonin	50–100 IU SC or IM daily, or 3 times/wk of salmon calcitonin 0.5 mg SC or IM daily or 2–3 times/wk of human calcitonin	Skin test before initial dose Side effects include nausea, vomiting, anorexia, flushing of palms of hands and soles of feet, urinary frequency Take at bedtime to minimize side effects Teach how to administer injections Assure adequate intake of calcium and Vitamin D

TABLE 7.4 (Continued)

Drug	Dose	Nursing Implications and Patient Teaching
Calcitonin nasal spray (Miacalcin) Approved in 1995	200–400 IU given in daily doses Alternate nares daily (right one day and left the next day)	Skin test before initial dose Side effects include mild nasal discomfort and rhinitis Contraindicated in clients who are allergic to injectable calcitonin Assure adequate intake of calcium and Vitamin D
Alendronate sodium (Fosamax) Approved in 1995	10 mg/d PO (treatment) 5 mg/d PO (prevention)	To ensure absorption, take with 6–8 oz. of water 30–90 minutes before first food or beverage of the day Take on an empty stomach Client must remain upright for 1 hr after taking Side effects include gastric distress, esophagitis, headache
Risedronate (Actonel) Approved in 2000	5 mg/d PO	Side effects include gastric distress Take with a full glass of water and remain upright 30 minutes prior to taking any other fluid or any food May be taken between meals or prior to bedtime Encourage adequate intake of calcium and Vitamin D but not to be taken at same time as Actonel
Selective Estrogen Receptor Modulator (SERMs)		
Raloxifene (Evista) Approved in 1998	60 mg/d PO	Can be taken without regard to time of day or meals Encourage adequate calcium and Vitamin D Contraindicated in women with history of DVT, pulmonary emboli or retinal vein thrombosis Highly protein bound Hot flashes may occur

Adapted from A. Maher, S. Salmond, T. Pellino, 1998, *Orthopaedic Nursing* (2nd ed.). Philadelphia: Saunders.

Estrogen replacement therapy

ERT has been shown to reduce the rate of trabecular bone loss and decrease the rate of fractures. Additionally, estrogen provides cardiovascular benefits and improves cognition. Estrogen replacement therapy should be started within three years of menopause. Adding progesterone can reduce the risk of endometrial cancer. The use of estrogen in treating women over age 70 with osteoporosis has not been clearly proven to be effective (Gamble, 1995a; Taxel, 1998).

Bisphosphonates

Bisphosphonates work by inhibiting bone resorption.

Calcitonin. Calcitonin is available in an injectable form or in a nasal spray. This medication works by inhibiting action of the osteoclasts leading to a slowed bone resorption. Calcitonin also has analgesic properties that help to relieve the pain of vertebral fractures (Taxel, 1998).

Alendronate (Fosamax®). Alendronate inhibits osteoclastic activity, leading to a decrease in bone resorption. It is the only drug that is recommended for both the treatment of (10 mg per day), and the prevention of (5 mg per day) osteoporosis (Taxel, 1998).

Risedronate (Actonel®). This drug is a third generation bisphosphonate and is more potent than earlier bisphosphonates, but has a reduced side effect profile. It inhibits osteoclastic activity. It is recommended that 5 mg per day be taken for long-term use (Kessenich, 2000).

Selective Estrogen Receptor Modulators (SERMs)

Raloxifene (Evista®). Raloxifene is the first selective estrogen receptor modulator approved for the treatment of osteoporosis. This class of drugs acts like estrogen in some parts of the body but not in others. Raloxifene increases BMD and also has beneficial cardiovascular effects, including decreasing cholesterol levels. This drug may also be protective against cancer of the breast (Kessenich, 1998).

NURSING MANAGEMENT

Because of the potential risks of osteoporosis and the high incidence of this disease, nurses have a responsibility to educate young people on prevention strategies. Middle-aged women should be advised to modify their lifestyle to potentiate bone remodeling. Older women who have osteoporosis should be taught how to best live with the disease and prevent injury and serious disability.

The following nursing diagnoses would be appropriate for the patient with osteoporosis:

- Altered nutrition, less than body requirements related to decreased calcium and Vitamin D intake
- Risk for injury related to weakened bone structure
- Impaired physical mobility related to weakness
- Pain related to acute/chronic effects of fracture
- Risk for altered health maintenance related to lack of knowledge of needed lifestyle changes
- Ineffective coping related to body image changes
- Anxiety related to fear of falling
- Risk for social isolation

Interventions and Outcomes

Altered nutrition, less than body requirements related to decreased calcium and Vitamin D intake

Expected outcome: The patient will state needed amounts of calcium and Vitamin D in the diet.

Nursing Interventions

- Instruct the patient on foods high in calcium (see Table 7.5)
- Instruct the patient on amounts of calcium supplements and the need to take in divided doses and with food for the best absorption.
- Instruct that Vitamin D can be obtained when the hands and face are exposed to 15–20 minutes of sunlight per day.
- Recommend lactose-free products if milk and milk products are not well tolerated.
- Instruct the patient that excessive calcium can lead to the development of kidney stones.

Dowd & Cavalieri, 1999; Galworthy & Wilson, 1996; Ignatavicius et al., 1999); Osteoporosis: A silent thief, 2000; Van Dyke et al., 2000).

TABLE 7.5 Dietary Sources of Calcium

Food	Calcium (mg)
Milk	
Skim milk, 1 cup	302
2% milk, 1 cup	297
Whole milk, 1 cup	291
Cheese	
Swiss cheese, 1 oz	272
Cheddar cheese, 1 oz	204
Processed American cheese,1 oz	174
Cottage cheese, 1oz	135
Lowfat yogurt, 8 oz	415
Ice cream, vanilla, 1 cup	176
Seafood	
Oysters, raw, 1 cup	226
Salmon, red, 3 oz, with bone	167
Vegetables	
Collards, 1 cup	357
Broccoli, 1 cup, fresh	177
Broccoli, 1 cup, frozen	94
Spinach, 1 cup	167
Dried bean (cooked, drained)	
Navy beans, 1 cup	90
Pinto beans, 1 cup	86
Red kidney beans, 1 cup	74
Peanuts, 1 cup	107

Adapted from "Osteoporosis: A Silent Thief," 2000, Dannemiller Memorial Education Foundation and Ventiv Health Communications [Monograph], 1–24.

Risk for injury related to weakened bone structure

Expected outcome: The patient will not experience a fall or accident that will result in fracture.

Nursing Interventions

- Teach the patient about safety and fall precautions, including the following:
  1. Avoid throw rugs but if used, make sure they are anchored with nonskid rubber backing.

2. Install grab bars in the bathroom along the tub/shower and beside the toilet.
3. Keep home free of clutter in walkways, including electrical cords and telephone wires.
4. Wear nonskid slippers and shoes.
5. Get up slowly after lying or sitting to prevent orthostatic hypotension.
6. Keep a nightlight on between the bedroom and bathroom.
7. Have adequate lighting throughout the house.

- Assess the patient's risk for falls whether the patient is in the home or long-term care.
- Assess the need for a cane or walker.
- Teach the patient not to lift heavy objects and to use good body mechanics.
- Assess for side effects of medications taken.
- Assess for other risk factors including use of alcohol, balance and gait problems, sensory problems, cognitive changes.
- Teach that golf and tennis may put an individual at risk for vertebral fracture though it may be safe to limit golf to putting.

(Dowd & Cavalieri, 1999; Galworthy & Wilson, 1996; Ignatavicius et al., 1999; Maher et al., 1998; Peterson, 2001; Van Dyke et al., 2000).

Impaired physical mobility related to weakness

Expected outcome: The patient will be able to participate in a regular exercise program.

Nursing Interventions

- Consult with physical therapy for a program of exercise and muscle strengthening.
- Encourage ROM exercises, which aid in joint mobility and improving muscle tone.
- Teach about the importance of weight-bearing exercise, such as walking, or bicycling, in maintaining bone mass.
- Teach that jogging and other vigorous activity provide too much stress on vertebrae.

- Recommend 30–60 minutes of exercise 3–4 times a week but any amount of exercise is better than none at all.
- Assess the need for assistive devices for performing ADLs.

(Dowd & Cavalieri, 1999; Galworthy & Wilson, 1996; Ignatavicius et al., 1999; Maher et al., 1998; Peterson, 2001; Van Dyke et al., 2000; Whipple, 1995).

Pain related to acute/chronic effects of fracture

Expected outcome: The patient will express a pain level of 2 or less on a 10-point scale *or* the patient will express an ability to maintain ADLs without pain or with minimal pain.

- Teach about taking medications for osteoporosis as ordered.
- Teach that pain may be managed with acetaminophen, anti-inflammatory medications, or stronger analgesics if necessary.
- Consult with physician on the efficacy of analgesics.
- Teach about outpatient therapy for heat and massage. For an acute vertebral fracture, ice and cool packs in the first 24–48 hours can assist in pain relief.
- Teach the client to avoid back flexion

(Dowd & Cavalieri 1999; Galworthy & Wilson, 1996; Ignatavicius, et al., 1999; Maher et al., 1998; Van Dyke et al., 2000).

Risk for altered health maintenance related to lack of knowledge of needed lifestyle changes

Expected outcome: The patient will state how lifestyle should be modified to help reduce incidence of increased bone demineralization.

Nursing Interventions

- Teach the patient about the disease and current treatment.
- Inform the patient about the National Osteoporosis Foundation.

- Teach the patient that tobacco should be reduced due to its toxic effects on bone and its effect on reduction of estrogen.
- Recommend a smoking cessation program.
- Teach that more than two drinks per day may reduce bone mass.
- Encourage a decrease in caffeine which has been shown to promote calcium loss through the urine.
- Teach the importance of BMD testing for all individuals 65 and older and those younger than 65 with risk factors or a previous fracture.
- Recommend a mediset container for taking medications prescribed for osteoporosis including calcium.

(Dowd & Cavalieri, 1999; Galworthy & Wilson, 1996; Ignatavicius et al., 1999; Maher et al., 1998; McClung, 2000; Peterson, 2001; Van Dyke et al., 2000).

Ineffective coping related to body image changes

Expected outcome: The patient will engage in activities that promote effective coping related to body image.

Nursing Interventions

- Provide information on osteoporosis support groups.
- Encourage the use of supportive undergarments with front closures.
- Recommend clothing such as mock turtlenecks, jackets and scarves, which de-emphasize the physical symptoms (kyphosis).
- Teach that physical therapists can assist with exercises to aid in improving posture.

(Dowd & Cavalieri, 1999; Galworthy & Wilson, 1996; Maher et al., 1998, Peterson, 2001; Van Dyke et al., 2000).

Anxiety related to fear of falling

Expected outcome: The patient will express a decrease in anxiety regarding falls.

Nursing Interventions

- Assure patients that their condition can be improved.
- Reinforce a positive attitude in patients and family members.
- Assess for need of assistive devices.
- Encourage the patient to walk normally rather than with slow, shuffling steps.
- Walk with the patient initially to assess abilities and reinforce that exercise will provide the needed strength to prevent falls.
- Teach the patient that inactivity contributes to bone demineralization and fracture risk.
- Encourage weight lifting and stretching which can strengthen the back.
- Encourage balance training such as yoga and tai chi can help in preventing falls.

(Dowd & Cavalieri, 1999; Galworthy & Wilson, 1996; Ignatavicius et al., 1999; Maher et al., 1998; Peterson, 2001)

Risk for social isolation

Expected outcome: The patient will continue to be involved in social activities.

Nursing Interventions

- Encourage the patient to become engaged in self-management of the disease.
- Discuss how the disease can lead to social withdrawal and depression.
- Encourage family members to assist the patient in maintaining social contacts when mobility becomes affected.
- Encourage modification of the living environment as needed to improve the quality of life.
- Allow the patient to verbalize the psychosocial effects the disease has had.

(Bayles, Cochran & Anderson, 2000; Galworthy & Wilson, 1996; Ignatavicius et al., 1999)

SUMMARY

Whether the patient is in the home, hospital, or long-term care setting, the nurse can provide valuable information and support to the patient with osteoporosis. The patient needs to be able to describe and implement the ordered treatment regimen to deal with this disease, including medications, diet, and lifestyle changes. For younger individuals at risk for the disease, nurses can help identify strategies for prevention so that their quality of life can be maintained as they age.

REFERENCES

Bayles, C., Cochran, K., & Anderson, C. (2000). The psychosocial aspects of osteoporosis in women. *Nursing Clinics of North America, 35*(1), 279–286.

Dannemiller Memorial Education Foundation and Ventiv Health Communications. (2000). *Osteoporosis: a silent thief.* Monograph, 1–24. The Author.

Dowd, R., & Cavalieri, J. (1999). Help your patient live with osteoporosis: Identifying risk, managing pain, overseeing treatment. *American Journal of Nursing, 99*(4), 55–60.

European Foundation for Osteoporosis and the National Osteoporosis, Foundation Consensus Development Statement. (1997). Who are candidates for prevention and treatment for osteoporosis?. *Osteoporosis International, 7*, 1–6.

Galsworthy, T., & Wilson, P. (1996). Osteoporosis: it steals more than bone. *American Journal of Nursing, 96*(6), 27–33.

Gamble, C. (1995a). Osteoporosis: making the diagnosis in patients at risk for fracture. *Geriatrics, 50*(7), 24–33.

Gamble, C. (19956). Osteoporosis: drug and nondrug therapies for the patient at risk. *Geriatrics, 50*(8), 39–43.

Hunt, A. (1996). The relationship between height change and bone mineral density. *Orthopaedic Nursing, 15*(3), 57–71.

Ignatavicius, D., Workman, M., & Mishler, M. (1999). *Medical-surgical nursing across the health care continuum.* (3rd ed.). Philadelphia: Saunders.

Kessenich, C. (1998). Raloxifene: a new class of anti-estrogens for the prevention of osteoporosis. *Nurse Practitioner, 23*(9), 91–93.

Kessenich, C. (2000). Risedronate: a new bisphosphonate for the treatment of osteoporosis. Nurse *Practitioner, 23*(3), 106–108.

Leslie, M. (2000). Issues in the nursing management of osteoporosis. *Nursing Clinics of North America, 35*(1), 189–197.

Maher, A., Salmond, S., & Pellino, T. (1998). *Orthopaedic nursing* (2nd ed.). Philadelphia: Saunders.

McClung, B., & Sieber, A. (2000). Clinical management of patients at risk for or diagnosed with osteoporosis. *Nursing Practice Guide, Medical Information Services,* 3–10.

National Osteoporosis Foundation. (1998). *Physician's guide to prevention and treatment of osteoporosis.* Washington DC: The Author.

National Resource Center. (2000). *Osteoporosis and related bone diseases: fast facts on osteoporosis.* Washington DC: The Author.

Peterson, J. (2001). Osteoporosis overview. *Geriatric Nursing, 22*(1), 17–21.

Schoen, D. (2000). *Adult orthopaedic nursing.* Philadelphia: Lippincott.

Taxel, P. (1998). Osteoporosis: detection, prevention, and treatment in primary care. *Geriatrics, 53*(8), 22–40.

Van Dyke Lamb, K., & Cummings, M. (2000). Musculoskeletal function. In A. Lueckenotte (Ed.), *Gerontologic Nursing* (2nd ed., pp. 740–744). St. Louis: Mosby.

Whipple, B. (1995). Common questions about osteoporosis and menopause. *American Journal of Nursing, 95*(1), 69–70.

WHO Study Group. (1994). *Assessment of fracture risk and its application to screening for postmenopausal osteoporosis. WHO Technical Report Series, no. 843.* Geneva, Switzerland: World Health Organization, 1–129.

PART II
Managing Arthritis

8
Assessing and Managing Pain

Ann Schmidt Luggen

The pain associated with arthritis is very complex. The term *arthritis* means joint inflammation, but significant inflammation is not a component of all types of arthritis. Although the source of pain is different in the different types of arthritis (Beherends, 1999), pain is frequently the most common symptom in older adults with all types of arthritis.

Arthritis pain may be chronic, acute, intermittent, and/or related to physical activity or weather. It is one of the most common symptoms for which elders consult their primary care providers. In arthritis, pain can be a major cause of disability, depression, loss of independence, isolation—all negative determinants in quality of life.

DEFINITION AND DESCRIPTION

Pain is often described as an unpleasant sensory and emotional experience associated with actual or perceived tissue damage. It is highly subjective even when the specific cause of pain is quite clear.

Acute Pain

This pain is of sudden onset, the etiology is often known, and the intensity may be severe. Examples of acute pain include a new fracture, a sprain, or a diagnostic procedure such as a biopsy.

Chronic Pain

This is long-lasting pain, months to years. The etiology may be unclear. Arthritis pain is frequently called chronic nonmalignant pain, which distinguishes it from cancer pain, another common cause of pain in elders. In both types of pain, the pain can become "the disease" (Katz, 2000).

CAUSES OF ARTHRITIS PAIN

Osteoarthritis

OA is characterized by degeneration of joint cartilage, which is the cushion at the point of articulation of two bones. Joint spaces contain synovial fluid that lubricates during joint motion. The cartilage thins and develops irregular surfaces. Osteophytes form at the joint margins. Small pieces of bone and cartilage float in synovial fluid (Irwin, 1999). At first, the pain is a dull ache with joint use. Rest relieves the pain. Stiffness is present on morning awakening. This lasts less than 30 minutes and diminishes with use. After years and continued degeneration, there is pressure and irritation of nerves. Soft tissue surrounding the joint becomes swollen. This becomes more painful than the joint pain. Now pain is present at rest, activity becomes limited, and joint stiffness is present even after use and activity.

Pain of Rheumatoid Arthritis

RA is caused by the deposition of immune complexes in the affected joints. This creates an inflammatory response that causes proteolytic enzyme formation, damaging the articular cartilage (Irwin, 1999). The joint inflammation is the source of pain, which increases over time. Synovitis occurs with congestion and edema of the synovial membrane and joint capsule. Pannus (thick layers of granulation tissue) forms, invading the cartilage and destroying the joint capsule and bone. Fibrous invasion of the pannus and subsequent scar formation occlude the joint space. Bone deteriorates and becomes misaligned. Disrupted joint articulation occurs with visible deformity. Fibrous tissue calcifies, resulting in total immobility

PATHOPHYSIOLOGY

Joint nerves contain many unmyelinated afferent axons(C-fibers) and few myelinated ones (A-fibers) (Willis, 2000). Thin C-fibers conduct slow, chronic pain. In contrast, thick A-fibers conduct nerve impulses from node to node in a fast, jumping manner and that transmits sharp, acute pain. These nerve fibers respond little to mechanical stimulation. However, they are greatly sensitized by inflammation and then will respond to even slight movement of the joint (allodynia).

As soft tissue becomes involved in arthritis progression, pain originates from deep tissues such as muscles. This pain may be referred (perceived) to the body wall. This occurs because of convergence of afferent nerve input from nociceptors (pain receptors) in the body wall and in deep tissue onto the same area of the spinal cord. Cartilage is not innervated and despite extensive destruction, does not cause pain.

INFLAMMATORY RESPONSE

Some of the factors responsible for the inflammatory response in arthritis are (Goldenberg, 2001):

- Prostaglandins
- Cytokines
- TNF-alpha
- IL-1beta
- Serotonin
- Bradykinin
- Norepinephrine
- Substance P

The identification of these factors has allowed scientists to discover modulators for treatment of rheumatologic diseases and their symptoms.

As disease progresses, nerve fibers become ever more sensitive, causing a secondary hyperalgesia, or an exaggerated pain response to a pain stimulus. A persistent nociception (somatic pain reception) develops and enlarges in area. New pain synapses are created with chemical and cellular changes that become permanent (Goldenberg, 2001).

ASSESSMENT OF ARTHRITIS PAIN IN OLDER ADULTS

Older adults present special considerations in pain assessment (Luggen, 1998). Long-lasting pain is often considered normal with aging and the older adult may not think to mention it to health professionals unless prodded. The author suggests that practitioners ask patients about discomfort rather than pain because older adults conceptually identify pain stimuli differently than younger adults. They are reluctant to label a painful stimulus as pain (Harkins & Chapman, 1977).

Other factors to consider in pain assessment in older adults include the complexity of the chronic painful problems that frequently occur concomitantly in older patients (Luggen, 1998). In a new patient assessment, it can be difficult to sort out new pain from other preexistent chronic illnesses. Further, quality of life issues need to be evaluated as there is a multidimensional relationship between pain and physical and functional well being, psychological well being, and social and spiritual well being (Ferrell, Phiner, Cohen, & Grant, 1991 and see Chapter 11 on quality of life).

Cultural Awareness

Our society is rapidly changing as it increases in diversity of age, races, cultures, and religions. Cultural diversity affects care of patients with pain. Patients undergoing similar procedures, such as knee aspiration, may have varied responses due to cultural differences. Pain is perceived in all cultures, differently in many cultures, and is perceived through the context of past experience with pain, spiritual beliefs, and religious beliefs about the meaning of pain.

There are biological differences among cultural groups, also. Neurological responses vary. Patients who have a genetic alteration in drug-metabolism (5–10% of the U.S. population) are unable to metabolize codeine to morphine and there is then no response to codeine (Showalter, 1999).

A frequently used assessment tool, the McGill Pain Questionnaire, assesses quality and intensity of pain in three dimensions: sensory, affective, and evaluative. This tool has been translated into several languages and is used in cross-cultural research (Showalter, 1999).

Coping

The coping mechanisms used throughout life need to be assessed. Older adults with pain may sometimes perceive pain as deserved or punishment from God for past wrongdoing or sins. In such cases, prayer may be used as a coping strategy. It may indicate giving up an active role in pain management and putting relief "into God's hands". Useful adaptive coping strategies can be encouraged. However, deep-rooted perceptions of the meaning of pain that are maladaptive are difficult to change.

Memory Loss

The status of memory must be assessed when obtaining a pain history in the older adult. It will be difficult to determine pain over the course of even 24 hours with some older patients. Family or caregiver assistance will be vital in this instance.

Cognitive impairment

Loss of cognition can present a major challenge to assessment. There has been considerable research on pain assessment in cognitively impaired elders in recent years and with the consistent use of simple popular pain instruments such as the "faces" pain scale, a tool used to assess pain in young children, most cognitively impaired patients can be assessed. One should try a number of tools to see which one is best understood by the individual client and then consistently use that one. A number of the most popular tools used in clinical practice today are identified in Box 8.1.

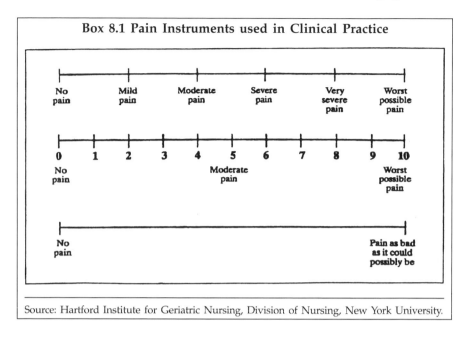

Box 8.1 Pain Instruments used in Clinical Practice

Source: Hartford Institute for Geriatric Nursing, Division of Nursing, New York University.

Gender Differences in Pain

Chronic pain is prevalent in about one in five Americans, and one in four of those older than 60 years of age (Katz, 2000). The prevalence of arthritis is greater in women than in men. Women are twice as likely as men to complain of pain and this tendency increases with age, especially in those older than 60.

Women may respond differently to pain medications than men. One study found that male rats required ten times more of a certain pain reliever than female rats in order to achieve the same analgesic effect (Essig, 2000). This points out the need to treat each client as an individual during assessment and management of pain.

Depression and Pain

Depression is not uncommon in older adults, and depression often accompanies pain in any individual, especially those suffering chronic pain, often called the cycle of pain. Depression is especially prevalent in nursing home settings. Assessment and management of depression becomes very important in pain management. There are many depression scales that are easy to use in any setting. Among them are (Sunderland, 1998):

- Geriatric depression scale
- NIMH dementia mood assessment scale (National Institutes of Mental Health)
- Zung Depression Scale
- Beck Depression Scale

Functional Ability

Mobility and independence must be assessed as a baseline and then periodically and over time as disease progression occurs. A primary dysfunctional method patients use to cope with arthritis pain is to decrease mobility and avoid pain. Evaluate Activities of Daily Living (ADLs) and Independent Activities of Daily Living (IADLs), and ambulation. Assess factors that contribute to or help alleviate pain. (see chapter 9 physical therapy). Functional status can be significantly enhanced with aggressive pain management.

Physical and Neurological Assessment

A comprehensive examination of the musculoskeletal and nervous system is needed. Identify affected joints, progression, changes, new joints, swelling, heat, redness and pain. Assess for trigger points. Conduct maneuvers that reproduce pain such as range of motion or straight leg raises. Movement should never be continued past the point of pain.

The neurological examination will focus on signs of sensory, motor, and autonomic deficits, looking for signs of nerve injury, for example, from compression from bony protruberances. A common example is sciatica, pain that radiates down one or both legs. This is neuropathic pain, or radiculopathy, which in many cases requires braces, surgical intervention, and/or different kinds of pharmaceutical intervention than traditional pain medications.

Specific Evaluation Areas

Assess for pain in each of the following upper extremity joints including hands, wrists, elbows, and shoulders. Evaluate each joint separately and compare with the opposite side. Many conditions affect the hands and wrists. There are more articulations in this area than any other (Katz, 2000). At a glance, one can see deformity and swelling. With a painful shoulder, most upper-extremity ADLs become lost. Simple activity such as brushing hair, or putting on a sweater or coat becomes too painful. Throwing a ball becomes impossible. Assess flexion, extension, pronation, supination, adduction, and abduction.

Knees

The knees should be carefully evaluated for swelling (effusion), tenderness, pain on movement, muscle wasting, deformity (enlargement), decreased range of motion, and most important, stability. Elders with knee problems often avoid pain by sitting for long periods and avoiding exercise, increasing the possibility of deconditioning. When deconditioning is evident, there is a great likelihood of falling.

Hips

Pain on movement is common in hip arthritis as is limitation of movement, especially on internal rotation. The joint may fix due to osteophyte formation of the femoral head and acetabulum. Like knee pain, severe hip pain usually limits the elder's willingness to exercise and bear weight and increases the risk of deconditioning.

Pain Assessment

Numerous tools are available and are seen in Box 8.1, p. 114. The 0–10 verbal scale is the most easily used in clinical practice. It is used to identify the intensity or level of pain and then check for pain relief.

The visual analogue scale (VAS) can be vertical or horizontal; the vertical is preferred by many older adults. The verbal rating scale is preferred over the VAS in one study of arthritis pain measurement (Langley & Sheppeard, 1984).

The word descriptor scale is used for qualitative measurement of pain and the faces scale is a graphic scale often used with children, but useful in older adults with cognitive impairment. In addition, it is helpful to periodically use the body scale (Box 8.2) to demonstrate where the pain is, where it is better, and any new pain. Some cogni-

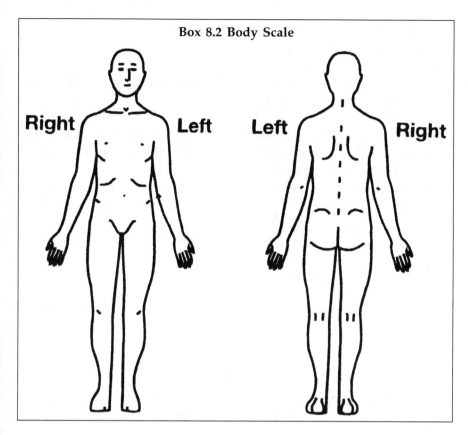

Box 8.2 Body Scale

tively impaired elders can point to the area of their bodies to show where pain is.

Whether or not pain scales are available, there are a number of specific questions to ask. These (and the scales if available) are:

- Onset-when the pain first started, when does daily onset occur
- Frequency-how often the patient experiences the pain
- Time of occurrence-for example, morning, evening, after exercise
- Location and radiation to other sites (use the body figure scale)
- Duration—how long the pain lasts
- Migration—ask about pain (radiates and moves around) and other related symptoms, stiffness

- Quality (use the word descriptor scale)
- Intensity (0–10 scale)
- Aggravating factors such as rain, cold weather
- Alleviating factors such as rest, immobility, pain medications, elevating an extremity, over-the-counter drugs, herbals

Further, it is useful to ask how the pain and stiffness interfere with daily life. This information gives the practitioner a sense of the meaning of arthritis in the patient's life.

The WOMAC Index (Western Ontario & McMaster Osteoarthritis Index) measures pain and function. It is frequently used in clinical trials to test therapies for arthritis.

Diagnostic tools include laboratory and imaging studies. However, radiography has not been found to correlate with elders' symptoms. Thirty percent of asymptomatic patients have radiographic abnormalities (Katz, 2000). Assessment of pain requires an analysis of all factors. The subjective complaints of the patient must be respected despite the presence or absence of objective findings.

MANAGEMENT: NURSING AND MEDICAL IMPLICATIONS

The goals of therapy for arthritis are

- Pain relief to increase function
- Reduction of swelling and inflammation to prevent further joint deterioration
- Protection from further injury, which may require splints to rest acute painful inflammation, or proper shoes
- Weight loss
- Avoidance of weight bearing during acute painful phases
- Anti-inflammatory analgesics

Prevention of disease progression includes managing pain so that progressive exercises can occur. Immobility of a joint due to pain can be a severe problem.

Medication Management

Management is based on a pyramid approach to managing pain, similar to the World Health Organization's model for management of cancer pain (WHO, 1990). Acetaminophen and NSAIDs (non-steroidal anti-inflammatory drugs) are most frequently used to treat arthritis, either alone in early disease or concomitantly with other medications.

Acetaminophen

According to the American College of Rheumatology guidelines for management of hip and knee OA (Brandt, 2000), acetaminophen is the first-line drug. *The Merck Manual of Geriatrics* (Beers & Berkow, 2000) also states that acetaminophen is the analgesic of choice for mild to moderate musculoskeletal pain in elders. Doses of 2600–4000 mg/day are effective in reducing arthritis pain. This drug provides analgesia but does not decrease inflammation. Doses are limited to 4 grams/day. Attention to the addition of acetaminophen in other medications, especially those over the counter, should be evaluated to keep the dose within this limit. Some prescribed drugs, such as Tylenol #3, contain acetaminophen.

Side effects of acetaminophen are usually mild and uncommon. Overdose can cause hepatotoxicity (AST>1000 u/L) and even hepatic failure with doses greater than 10 gm. Increased alcohol intake increases the risk of liver toxicity if the dose is exceeded (Brandt, 2000). Chronic use of acetaminophen can increase the risk of chronic renal disease. However, a cause/effect relationship here is not conclusive. Some clinicians have prescribed aspirin in place of acetaminophen in elders with renal failure; however, the complications with aspirin on platelets, the GI mucosa, and renal blood flow preclude its use (Brandt). Further, the National Kidney Foundation's position paper states that acetaminophen continues as the non-narcotic analgesic of choice for episodic use in patients with underlying renal disease (Brandt).

Warfarin (Coumadin) is potentiated by acetaminophen (Brandt, 2000). Patients taking four 325 mg tablets/day for more than one week have a 10 times greater risk of an INR greater than 6 (laboratory test indicating possibility of hemorrhage). An intervention is warranted for an INR greater than 3.5 to 4. The risk of hemorrhage decreases with lowered doses of acetaminophen.

Box 8.3 Monitoring NSAIDs
Hematocrit
Hemoglobin
Occult blood in stool

NSAIDs

These drugs are indicated for short-term use in inflammatory arthritis conditions (Beers & Berkow, 2000). NSAIDs are not all the same. If one NSAID is not effective, it does not predict response to another. NSAIDs have a ceiling effect, that is, there is a level of efficacy at which increasing the dose does not result in an increased analgesic effect.

The adverse effects of NSAIDs are very high in older adults. The risk of gastrointestinal (GI) bleed is at least 10% in those older than 60 years of age who have a history of GI bleed in the past (see Box 8.3).

Other GI adverse effects are also high when using NSAIDs. In two major trials of three NSAIDs, GI adverse effects were 18.7%, 15.4%, and 13.3% (Brandt, 2000). NSAIDs consistently rating high in GI toxicity are piroxicam, ketoprofen, and tolmectin. Other NSAIDs that older adults should avoid are indomethacin, which has central nervous system (CNS) side effects, and meclofenamate, which causes diarrhea.

Some GI effects can be reduced with misoprostol, although this use is controversial (Brandt, 2000). Further, misoprostol is expensive, does not decrease the side effect of dyspepsia, and frequently has the side effect of diarrhea. H2 receptor antagonists and proton pump inhibitors are known to be effective in treatment and prevention of NSAID-induced ulcers (Brandt).

NSAIDs produce an analgesic effect in about one hour and the effect lasts six to eight or more hours. The anti-inflammatory effects may take two to three weeks to occur and last two to four weeks (Montgomery, 1999).

Drug interactions with NSAIDs are common. NSAIDs are highly plasma protein bound. Drug interactions often include (but do vary within the NSAID class of drugs)

- Aspirin—increases risk of GI bleed
- Methotrexate-a commonly used drug for RA, potentiates toxicity

- Lithium-increases lithium levels
- Acetaminophen—increases 50% the acetaminophen plasma levels
- Anticoagulants-increase the anticoagulant effect, increasing risk of bleeding
- Phenytoin-increases toxicity
- Beta blockers, diuretics, and ACE inhibitors-decrease the antihypertensive effects

COX-2 Inhibitors

COX-2 produces pain-producing prostaglandins in response to injury or inflammation. COX-2 inhibitors block this effect, allowing COX-1 to be present protects GI mucosa, platelet regulation, and maintenance of renal blood flow. Other NSAIDs block both COX-1 and COX-2.

Patients with arthritis are 2–1/2 to 5–1/2 times more likely to be hospitalized for NSAID-related GI toxicity with a cumulative risk over time (Katz, 2000). COX-2 inhibitors are believed to reduce this risk.

At the time of publication, two COX-2 inhibitors are available: Celecoxib (Celebrex©) and Rofecoxib (Vioxx©). Celecoxib has a ½ life of 11 hours (Katz 2000) and 2x/day dosing is recommended at 100–200 mg/dose. Celecoxib inhibits the cytochrome P450 isoenzyme 2D6 and may increase the effects of drugs metabolized by this enzyme, including beta blockers, tricyclic antidepressants, antiarrhythmics, ecainamide, and flecainide (Katz). Celecoxib contains sulfur and is contraindicated in those with sulfa allergy or allergy to aspirin or other NSAIDs. There has been no difference in safety or efficacy observed in older adults when compared to younger adults. Drug interactions are generally the same as NSAIDs. Celecoxib has FDA (Federal Drug Administration) approval for OA and RA pain.

Rofecoxib works similarly to celecoxib, blocking COX-2 and sparing COX-1, which protects the stomach lining. Rofecoxib is approved by the FDA for OA pain and for acute general pain.

Tramadol

This is a centrally acting analgesic, as are the opioids. It is not an NSAID, is opioid-like, and has low plasma protein binding. The liver metabolizes it. Tramadol is useful for moderate to severe pain as an analgesic; it is not an anti-inflammatory drug. It is effective for

OA, low back pain, peripheral neuropathy, and orthopedic and post-operative pain (Katz, 2000).

In elderly patients, the 'start low and go slow' adage is important. Slow introduction of Tramadol reduces the incidence of side effects of nausea, vomiting, and dizziness. Start at one-half the recommended dose of 50 mg (25 mg) in the morning, and every three days increase the dose until the patient is taking 25 mg qid. Then increase from 25 to 50 mg until the desired pain relief is achieved. It is not recommended that older adults, especially those greater than 75 take more than 300 mg/day (Katz, 2000).

Tramadol© can increase the risk of seizures in patients with epilepsy and with concomitant use of SSRIs (serotonin reuptake inhibitors), tricyclic antidepressants, and opioids (Katz, 2000). Side effects of Tramadol are considered a nuisance and not organ-damaging. It is considered a second-line drug after acetaminophen and before NSAIDs by many specialists (Katz). It is very useful for breakthrough pain in OA flashes when more pain control is needed. It is also useful in combination with NSAIDs in lower doses and with increased efficacy.

Opioids

These drugs relieve all types of arthritis pain. In older adults, they have a longer half life (Beers & Berkow, 2000) and have a greater analgesic effect as well (Baran, 2000).

When first given, opiods can cause drowsiness, cognitive impairment, and, occasionally, respiratory depression. This usually lasts just a few days until tolerance develops (Beers & Berkow, 2000). Precautions should be taken in terms of driving and falls during this period. For side effects of opiods and to monitor side effects of opioids see Box 8.4.

All opioid prescriptions should be accompanied by an anticonstipation regime. See Box 8.5 for foods that alleviate constipation. Constipation is a side effect of opioids that is not improved with tolerance to the drugs.

Opiates act centrally, blocking opioid receptor sites centrally and peripherally. Morphine is the prototype and standard against which all other analgesics are measured (Katz, 2000). Morphine is rarely used in treatment of arthritis, but less potent opioids are commonly prescribed.

Box 8.4 Monitoring Side Effects of Opioids

Sedation
Nausea
Constipation
Urinary retention
Mental clouding
Respiratory depression
Drowsiness
Gastroparesis
Colonic paresis

Oxycodone. Oxycodone is very useful in moderately severe, chronic painful arthritis. It is available in immediate and controlled-release forms and has fewer side effects than morphine. Side effects include nausea and vomiting, although less frequently than with morphine. As with most drugs in older adults, start low with opioids and increase slowly until the desired level of relief is achieved.

Fentanyl. Fentanyl, which is more potent than morphine, is sometimes prescribed for its convenience of a patch that needs renewal only every 3 days. This may be especially convenient for cognitively impaired elders who refuse to swallow food and medications. Moderately severe arthritis pain may be alleviated and allow good functioning with the fentanyl patch. The first dose does not reach peak analgesic effect for 18–24 hours after application.

Corticosteroids

These are used in some kinds of arthritis such as OA, RA, and gout as an adjunct to pain management and for improving function (see Box 8.6). The drugs should not be used frequently because of the tendency for chondrolysis. It is recommended that fewer than four times per year is safe and effective. Elders should not bear weight on the steroid-injected joint for three days post injection (Katz, 2000).

Box 8.5 Foods to Prevent Constipation

High fiber foods: oatmeal, bran, whole wheat, rye, apples, pears, beans, dry beans, peas, cabbage, root vegetables, fresh tomatoes, carrots, green beans, peaches, plums, strawberries, citrus.

*Adapted from Luggen (2000)

Box 8.6 Side Effects of High-dose, Long-term Use of Corticosteroids

- osteoporosis
- cataracts
- decreased wound healing
- hyperglycemia
- hypertension
- elevated lipids
- increased risk of infection

(Beers & Berkow, 2000).

Systemic corticosteroids are very effective in treating chronic inflammatory arthritis (Katz, 2000). There are serious side effects for elderly patients on high dose, long-term corticosteroids. Usually, low dose prednisone can achieve effective pain control at a dose of about 5 mg daily. This is useful for RA and PMR (polymyalgia rheumatica). It can be used in conjunction with NSAIDs but this increases the risk of GI complications.

Antidepressants

Because depression is frequently a component of chronic pain, this class of drugs may raise the pain threshold and reduce analgesia need, in addition to reducing depressed mood. Tricyclic antidepressants (TCAs) are usually given and may be most effective for this purpose; however, they are used less frequently in elderly patients than are SSRIs (selective serotonin reuptake inhibitors). The anticholinergic effects and central nervous system effects of TCAs may af-

---

Box 8.7 Anticholinergic and Other Effects of Tricyclic Antidepressants

- urinary retention
- constipation
- blurred vision
- dry mouth
- weight gain
- memory impairment
- sedation

(Katz, 2000).

TABLE 8.1 Drugs to Avoid in Pain Management of Older Adults

Drug	Precautions	Solutions
Meperidine (Demerol@)	Low oral potency Metabolite, may cause seizures, confusion, agitation	Choose drug with higher potency, another opiate
Pentazocine (Talwin@)	CNS excitement, confusion, and agitation	Avoid all use in elders
Propoxyphene (Darvon@)	Potency no better than ASA, signifi- cant abuse potential, renal injury potential	Use NSAID or weak opioid
Methadone (Dolophine@)	Very long half life	Use weak opioid

*Adapted from Luggen (2000).

fect balance, gait, and attention levels (Katz, 2000). Cardiovascular effects in patients with hypertension and cardiac disease preclude TCA use in these patients. Also, lowered renal clearance of the metabolites of TCAs requires further caution (Katz).

The advantages of SSRIs includes fewer side effects compared to TCAs. Fluoxetine (Prozac©) and paroxitine (Paxil©) are often used in elderly patients. They are nonsedating and have decreased incidence of cognitive dysfunction. Side effects do occur—nausea, anxiety, insomnia, and impaired sexual function. Many resolve in two to three weeks after treatment has begun. Patients are given one oral dose/day; some companies have developed once/week dosing. There are a number of drugs that should not be given to older adults as the side effects are problematic (see Table 8.1).

Non-Medication Pain Management

Our patients often know what helps to relieve pain. This is a part of the pain assessment. However, when patients are also depressed with pain, they may feel hopeless about obtaining pain relief. Many patients with arthritis think that medication is the mainstay of pain management (Campbell & Linc, 1999). However there are many other tools in our repertoire to manage pain. For a more extensive discussion of these methods, see chapter 9 on exercise and physical therapy, and chapter 12 on alternative and complementary therapies.

Cold

This is helpful in reducing inflammation and edema that cause pain. It may reduce muscle spasms that are associated with arthritis. Cold can be given via cold packs or ice bags (using caution), or cool soaks and baths.

Warmth

Many older adults with morning pain and stiffness will find relief from a warm bath or shower.

Exercise

In early arthritis, without inflammation, exercise can prevent stiffness, maintain function, relieve muscle spasm and increase the elder's sense of well being (Luggen, 2000). Analgesics may be needed prior to starting exercise. In late stage arthritis and with inflammation, the exercise program should be conducted in consultation with a rheumatologist (arthritis specialist) and a physical therapist.

Massage

Many forms of touch are pleasurable to older adults (Ebersole & Hess, 1998). Based on individual preference, massage may be rubbing, kneading with deep pressure, or light stroking and smooth stroking. In frail elders who may have severe osteoporosis, caution must rule. When combining massage with aromatherapy, individual preference for different odors or fragrances should be elicited.

Acupressure and Acupuncture

Manual pressure at specific acupuncture sites is acupressure. The insertion of needles at those sites with manual or electrical stimulation is acupuncture. The stimulation competes for placement on pain receptor sites stopping the progression of pain messages to higher brain centers (Luggen, 2000). This therapy is conducted by certified health professionals, often by nurses.

TENS

Transcutaneous electrical nerve stimulation (TENS) is useful in the management of pain in older adults. It consists of intermittent low voltage current applied to skin – noninvasive, few side effects, battery powered, can be worked by patients. Patients have control of the intensity of stimulation of the electrodes on the skin. TENS has had limited testing for arthritis in older adults and may be a consideration for research. It has been useful for neuropathic pain and spine pain (Eiman, Anderson, Donela, & Silverman, 1996).

Distractions

This method of modulation of pain perception can be almost anything, from reading a book to watching TV to entertaining guests. It takes one's attention from the feeling of pain. It is only useful for mild pain; moderate and moderately severe pain require analgesics in addition to the distraction. Music is a special type of distraction that has been used extensively in clinical practice with older adults (Clair, 1996). The type of music used should be appreciated or selected by the older adult and played at a volume that the elder can control.

Therapeutic Touch

Therapeutic touch (TT) is a pain management modality that is being used with increasing frequency in older adults. The therapy directs energy to the patient to give pain relief. The nurse therapist combines "compassionate intent" with hand movements that "rebalance" a person's energy (Hutchison, 1999). It is associated with "life energy" the Chinese *qi*. The therapist "centers," attaining a meditative state sensitive to the elder's needs. A balance of the person's energy levels (not too high, not too low) or harmony is the goal of therapy. (see chapter 12 on alternative therapies.)

SUMMARY

Arthritis is a group of diseases that increase in frequency in older adults world wide. They often assume the guise of simple aging and do not receive the attention that would aid in increasing the quality of life that is lost without that attention. There are many management modalities available to us as caregivers to this population. We can make a difference in the quality of life of our patients.

REFERENCES

Baran, R. W. (2000). Guidelines for the management of chronic nonmalignant pain in the elderly LTC resident: The relief paradigm, Part I. *LTC Clinical Interface*, Nov-Dec. (Booklet)

Beers, M. H. & Berkow, R. (Eds.). (2000). *The Merck manual of geriatrics* (3rd ed.). Whitehouse Station, NJ: Merck.

Beherends, J. (1999, September 9). Arthritis. http://adultpain.nursing.uiowa.edu

Brandt, K. D. (2000). *Diagnosis and nonsurgical management of OA* (2nd ed.). Caddo, OK: Professional Com. Inc.

Campbell, J. M. & Linc, L. G. (1999). Managing osteoarthritis pain: Strategies for elderly patients. *Advance for Nurse Practitioners, 7*(4); 57–60.

Clair, A. A. (1996). *Therapeutic uses of music with older adults*. Baltimore: Health Professions Press.

Ebersole, P. & Hess, P. (1998). *Toward healthy aging: Human needs and nursing response*. 5th ed. St. Louis: Mosby.

Eiman, A., Anderson, T., Donela, P., & Silverman, P. (1996). Geriatric pain management. In E. Salerno & J. Willens (Eds.). *Pain management handbook*. St. Louis: Mosby.

Essig, M. G. (2000, April 2). Men and women may respond differently to pain relievers. http://webmd-practice.medcast.com

Ferrell, B. R., Rhiner, M., Cohen, M., Grant, M., (1991). Pains as a metaphor for illness. *Oncology Nursing Forum, 8*(8); 1303-1309.

Goldenberg, D. L. (2001). Chronic pain management. In S. Ruddy, E. D. Hanes Jr. & C. B. Sledge (Eds.), *Kelley's textbook of rheumatology*, (pp. 753–762). Philadelphia: Sanders.

Harkins, S. & Chapman, C. (1977). The perception of induced dental pain in young and elderly women. *Journal of Gerontology, 32*(4); 428–435.

Irwin, C. (1999, September 9). Arthritis: why it hurts. http://adultpain.nursing.uiowa.edu

Katz, W. A. (2000). Pain management in rheumatic disorders. Drugsmartz Publ: U.S.

Langley G. B. & Sheppeard, H. (1984). Problems associated with pain measurement in arthritis: Comparison of the VA and VR scales. *Clinical and Experimental Rheumatology, 2*, 231–234.

Luggen A. (2000). Pain. In A. Lueckenotte (Ed.). *Gerontological nursing*, (pp. 281-301). St. Louis: Mosby.

Luggen, A. (1998). Chronic pain in older adults: A quality of life issue. *JOGN, 24*(2), 48–54.

Montgomery, J. (1999, September 19). Naproxen sodium. http://www Nursing.uiowa.edu.

Showalter, S. (1999, September 9). Culture and pain. http://adultpain. nursing.uiowa.edu.

Sunderland, T. (1998). A new scale for assessment of depressed mood in demented patients. *American Journal of Psychiatry*, 145, 955–957.

World Health Organization. (1990). *Cancer relief and palliative care: Report of a WHO expert committee*. Geneva: author.

Willis, W. D. (2000, May 26). Mechanisms of somatic pain. http://talaria.org.

9

Exercise and Physical Therapy

Barbara Resnick

Arthritis is a common chronic illness experienced by older adults. Almost half of all older adults have arthritis, and projections indicate that by 2020 almost 60 million individuals will have some evidence of arthritis ("Arthritis", 2000). Older adults who have arthritis are more likely to need help with personal care activities such as bathing, dressing, and toileting, as well as help with instrumental activities of daily living such as preparing meals, shopping, or using the telephone (National Institute of Arthritis and Musculoskeletal and Skin Disease, 1998). Individuals with arthritis also tend to report their health as fair or poor rather than excellent or very good, and these individuals have twice as many visits to a health care provider when compared to those without arthritis. Moreover, arthritis can result in social isolation and influence quality of life ("Arthritis", 2000). Health care providers and patients alike have reported that pain and loss of functioning are the most important problems individuals with arthritis face, and at this time there is no cure for this disease. There are, however, many treatment options in addition to medication management.

DISPELLING THE MYTHS RELATED TO ARTHRITIS ABOUT EXERCISE AND ACTIVITY

Many people believe that an arthritic joint should be left to rest, and that exercise and therapy only aggravate the problems of these joints and make the arthritis worse. Trauma and repetitive strenuous activities, such as playing football can promote osteoarthritis. There are many activities done in therapy, however, and well-planned exercise that will actually help joints. Regular activity, such as running and walking, has not been associated with the development of arthritis. Moreover, there is support to indicate that these activities may actually help with the management of the disease.

Prolonged inactivity because of osteoarthritis can result in poor aerobic capacity and increased risk for cardiovascular disease, obesity, and other inactivity-related disorders. Distention of the knee joint capsule because of fluid accumulation in osteoarthritis of the knee inhibits quadriceps muscular contraction, compounding the loss of strength in the quadriceps initiated by inactivity. There is also evidence that deconditioned muscle, inadequate motion, and stiffness around the joint may contribute to signs and symptoms of osteoarthritis (Slemenda et al., 1997).

Arthritis can have multiple effects on the musculoskeletal system including pain, swelling, decreased joint range of motion, muscle weakness, and instability. These problems lead to decreased activity and poor cardiovascular fitness. Many of these problems can actually stem from physical inactivity. Inactivity, and the adoption of a sedentary lifestyle due to arthritis may actually exacerbate the signs and symptoms of arthritis.

EXERCISE AND OSTEOARTHRITIS

Although many older adults with arthritis tend to avoid activity and exercise, exercise is actually one of the most effective nonpharmacologic treatments for osteoarthritis, particularly osteoarthritis of the knee (Deyle et al., 2000; S. H. Ettinger et al., 1994; W. H. Ettinger et al., 1997). Well-conditioned muscle and muscular balance are needed to withstand physical activity such as walking, provide joint stability, and support function and independence. Muscular conditioning can be achieved through well-designed exercise programs. Specifically, long-term walking (W. H. Ettinger et al., 1997; Messier, Thompson, & Ettinger, 1997), isokinetic quadriceps exercise (Hurley & Scott, 1998; O'Reilly, Muir, & Doherty, 1999; Maurer, Stern, Knossian, Cook, & Schumacher, 1999), high and low intensity bicycling (Mangione et al., 1999), aquatic exercise classes (Spencer, Kinne, Betza, Ramsey, & Patrick, 1998), and a 12–week program of specially designed physiotherapy improved physical function and gait, and reduced knee pain in older adults with arthritis (Van Baar et al., 1998). The Fitness Arthritis and Seniors Trial (FAST) (Messier et al., 2000) is the largest clinical trial to date that evaluated the effects of exercise on osteoarthritis. A total of 439 older adults were randomized to receive aerobic exercise, resistance exercise, or routine care (health education). The participants in the aerobic exercise group exercised for 40-minute three times a week, those in the resistance exercise group completed three 40-minutes sessions per week, performing two sets of 12 repetitions of nine exercises. The study results indicated that both aerobic walking and weight training improve postural sway and thereby improve balance and ambulation, and that physical disability and performance were improved and pain was reduced. The increasing number of studies demonstrating the benefits of exercise for older adults with osteoarthritis clearly indicate that aerobic and strength training exercises improve strength, exercise capacity, gait, functional performance, and balance, and decrease the risk of falling.

GOALS OF EXERCISE

The specific goals of exercise in osteoarthritis are to prevent deconditioning of the muscles that keep the joints stable, to improve joint flexibility, and to enhance aerobic fitness, while maintaining good joint protection. Muscles that do not get used regularly because of pain will atrophy. A comprehensive exercise program should therefore include stretching exercises, followed by a range-of-motion program for the affected joint, muscle strengthening, and aerobic exercise if possible (see Table 9.1). The exercise prescriptions are based on the physiologic principles of overload and specificity. The overload principle states that when a muscle or a group of muscles is subjected to

TABLE 9.1 Guidelines for Exercise Programs for Older Adults with Arthritis

Type of Exercise Activity	Specific Recommendations
Stretching	1. Should be done daily for 10 minutes and cover all muscle groups. 2. The individual should be encouraged to stretch to the point of mild discomfort, hold the stretch for 10 to 30 seconds, and repeat this 3 to 5 times.
Range of motion	1. Should put all joints through full range of motion daily.
Resistive	1. The intensity is manipulated by varying the weight, the number of repetitions, the length of the rest interval between exercises, and the number of sets (groups) of exercises completed. 2. Should be rhythmical, performed at moderate-to-slow speed, involve a full range of motion, and not interfere with breathing. 3. Perform three sets of eight to ten repetitions of the exercise. When able to do this easily the resistance should be increased (i.e., move from one to two pounds, for example).
Aerobic	1. Training should begin at low levels and gradually increase to 60 to 80% of maximal heart rate (MHR). To calculate 70% of MHR the formula 220–age x .70 is used. 2. Increasing the intensity of aerobic activity can be done by adding weights, going up hills, or simply increasing the pace of movement and adding more arm and leg movement.

physiologic stresses that exceed customary levels, adaptation and increased capacity occur. Overload can be accomplished by increasing the exercise intensity, duration, frequency, or a combination of these factors. The principle of specificity implies that improvements in musculoskeletal performance are determined by the method of training. For example, if the goal is to improve knee extensor strength, then exercises to increase quadriceps strength using some type of resistance would be recommended. Adequate joint motion and elasticity of tissues around the joint are necessary for cartilage nutrition and health, protection of joint structures from damaging impact loads, and function and comfort in daily activities. Range-of-motion exercises should be performed daily to maintain the joint range and prevent contractures. Appendix A (p. 154) provides a list of resources that have developed written exercise programs appropriate for individuals with osteoarthritis.

Stretching Exercise

Joint flexibility is essential and can help improve muscle performance, reduce the risk for injury, and improve cartilage nutrition. Exercise should be the first step in any program to improve flexibility. The main objectives of these stretching and range-of-motion exercises are to relieve joint stiffness, increase joint flexibility, and prevent soft tissue contractures by increasing the length and elasticity of the muscles and tissues around the joints. Joint range of motion can be started before or in conjunction with resistance and aerobic exercise programs.

Isometric Exercise

Older adults with arthritis often have a limited range of motion, especially in their lower extremities. It is often this decreased range of motion at the knee and hip that causes the pain, loss of function, and physical limitations associated with arthritis. Range of motion and isometric strengthening exercises, which are exercises that contract muscles without moving the joint, are very effective in decreasing pain and improving function, and less likely to exacerbate arthritis pain.

Extremely forceful muscle contractions will increase intra-articular pressure and may promote cartilage damage. Therefore, multiple repetitions at a lower intensity than the individual is capable of are optimal initially to prevent flares in disease. Isometric strengthening exercises, which are exercises that move the joint in an arc, can be gently performed against gravity resistance initially and then with progressive weights added as tolerated. If joint pain prevents movement through certain ranges, the range of motion of the strengthening exercise can be limited to the pain-free zone. Attempts should be made to extend the range of the joint until the full range of motion is covered; otherwise strength increases will be limited to the joint angles, or position, at which training is conducted. Ultimately it is muscle strengthening that will help support the osteoarthritic joint, decrease pain, and improve function.

Isotonic Exercise or Resistance Training

An isotonic muscle contraction is characterized by variable joint speed against a constant resistance (i.e., a weight). This type of exercise closely corresponds to everyday activities such as lifting groceries, and is strongly recommended for older adults with arthritis. Knowing the amount of resistance to use, and when to increase that resistance is based on the individual's ability. One repetition maximum is most commonly the measure used to make that determination. One repetition maximum (RM) is the maximum mass of free weight or other resistance that can be moved by a muscle group through the full range of motion using good form, one time. Good form is evident when the exercise is performed by the specific muscle group only. Generally, the patient is instructed to perform three sets of eight to ten repetitions of the exercise. When the patient is able to do this easily, the resistance should be increased (change from one to two pounds for example). To prevent acute flares older adults with osteoarthritis should not be pushed to add resistance (i.e., weights) beyond which they are easily capable of using.

Aerobic Exercise

Aerobic exercise, such as walking, is generally well tolerated in older adults with mild to moderate lower extremity osteoarthritis (Lane & Buckwalter, 1993; Messier et al., 2000). Low intensity exercise is defined as exercising at a heart rate of less than 60% of the individuals' maximum heart rate (220 - age), and moderate intensity exercise is at 60 to 80% of the maximum heart rate. Alternatively, exercise intensity may be based on the individuals' subjective report of psychological strain associated with the exercise activity, or his or her rate of perceived exertion (RPE) based on the Borg scale (Borg, 1982, see Table 9.2). To complete the Borg scale the individual is asked to rate, on a scale of 6 (very, very light exercise exertion) to 20 (very very hard exercise exertion) how they perceive their exercise work. A RPE score on the Borg measure between 12 and 16 correlates with

TABLE 9.2 Borg Perceived Exertion Scale

Numerical Scale	Ratings
6	
7	very very light
8	
9	very light
10	
11	fairly light
12	
13	somewhat hard
14	
15	hard
16	
17	very hard
18	
19	very very hard
20	

reaching 60 to 80% of the targeted heart rate, and assures that the individual is exercising at a moderate intensity.

Exercise prescriptions must consider the intensity, duration, frequency, and progression of exercise. Intensity, by definition, is the amount of effort or exertion put forth during the activity, and, as described above, can be measured using simple techniques such as the Borg Test. Training duration is how long the exercise is performed. For aerobic activity this is the amount of time the individual does the activity, and for resistive exercise it is the number of repetitions performed. Duration and intensity are inversely related to each other. That is, a more intense strengthening program requires fewer repetitions with increased amount of weight. Training frequency has to do with how many times a week the individual engages in the activity. The progression of any exercise program depends on the individual's response to exercise. For most older adults with arthritis there is usually a 2.5% increase per week in either the intensity or duration of exercise.

Unfortunately, for older adults with more severe osteoarthritis, walking to perform aerobic exercise may not be well tolerated. Alternative options are non-or partial weight-bearing aerobic exercise such as biking, swimming, water walking (i.e., walking in deep water), or upper extremity aerobic biking (i.e., pedaling with upper extremities). In some situations it may be necessary to begin with resistance training exercises before adding aerobic activity. The resistive exercises will stabilize the knee by increasing the strength of knee extensors, flexors, tendons, and ligaments around the joint and will ultimately reduce the pain so that the patient can tolerate weight-bearing aerobic activity.

Water Aerobics

Particularly for older adults who have significant pain with range of motion and weight bearing, an aquatic aerobic training program may be very therapeutic. In water, aquatic therapy practitioners use the buoyancy, viscosity, hydrostatic pressure, resistance and other unique properties of water. Because water provides a therapeutic environment much different than land, it is not recommended that therapists merely take land-based treatments and place them, unchanged, in the pool. It is much more typical for therapists to either significantly modify existing land-based treatments or to perform techniques that were specifically created to be used in water. Examples of some of these techniques are shown in Table 9.3.

EXERCISE FOR RHEUMATOID AND INFLAMMATORY ARTHRITIS

Although less extensively studied, exercise has been noted to decrease acute inflammation of joints, improve function, and decrease pain for individuals with rheumatoid or inflammatory arthritis. Static and dynamic shoulder rotator exercises in women with rheumatoid arthritis decreased the number of swollen joints in the upper extremities, and decreased shoulder pain (Bostrom, Harms-Ringdahl, Karreskog, & Nordemar, 1998). In a comprehensive review of studies that tested the impact of dynamic exercise on individuals with rheumatoid arthritis, Van den Ende, Vliet Vlieland, Munneke, and Hazes (1998), reported that dynamic exercise was effective in increasing aerobic capacity and muscle strength. Moreover, there were

TABLE 9.3 Examples of Aquatic Exercise Treatment for Arthritis

Technique	Description
Ai Chi	A form of active aquatic therapy or fitness modeled after the principles of T'ai Chi and yogic breathing techniques.
	Ai Chi is typically provided in a hands-off manner (the provider stands on the pool deck to allow visual imaging of complex patterns by the client). The client stands in chest-deep water and is verbally and visually instructed by the provider to perform a slow, rhythmic combination of therapeutic movements and deep breathing.
Proprioceptive neuromuscular facilitation	A form of active aquatic therapy modeled after the principles and movement patterns of Proprioceptive Neuromuscular Facilitation (PNF).
	Aquatic PNF can be provided in either a hands-on or hands-off manner.
	The client is verbally, visually, and/or tactilely instructed in a series of functional, spiral and diagonal, mass movement patterns while standing, sitting, kneeling or lying in the water. The patterns may be performed actively, or with assistance or resistance provided by specialized aquatic equipment or the provider.
Bad Ragaz	Bad Ragaz is always performed in a hands-on manner by the provider.
	The client is verbally, visually and/or tactilely instructed in a series of movement or relaxation patterns while positioned horizontally and supported by rings or floats in the water.
	The patterns may be performed passively (for flexibility and relaxation), actively, or with assistance or resistance from a provider.

no detrimental effects of exercise on disease activity, disease progression or pain.

Like noninflammatory arthritis or degenerative joint disease, exercise activity for those with inflammatory arthritis should include a warm-up period of gentle stretching to loosen muscles and tendons, range-of-motion exercises to move each joint carefully through its full range, muscle strengthening to strengthen and support joints, and aerobic activity to increase cardiovascular stamina. The exercises included should not, however, be performed with joints that are actively inflamed.

Stretching and Warm-up Exercises

Stretching and warm-up exercises are particularly important in inflammatory arthritis to prevent undue stress to inflamed muscle tendons that can tear in their weakened state. The joints should not be rapidly or ballistically (repetitive bouncing movements) stretched to their furthest degree. Rather, joint range-of-motion exercises should attempt to fully move the joint while supporting the joint and surrounding muscles. The opposite arm or leg may assist in this effort. Muscle strengthening, or resistance training, is not recommended for a severely inflamed joint. During acute inflammation, the joints should be moved gently through the fullest pain-free range of motion. During this acute inflammatory phase, a physical therapist should be involved to prevent overstretching of inflamed tissues and compromising joint stability. The application of cold prior to stretching may help to reduce the pain involved. However, once the acute episode resolves, muscle strengthening should be resumed to prevent muscle atrophy around inflamed joints. Moreover, *all* other joints and muscles should be exercised during a flare as strong muscles provide support to the damaged joints. It has been shown that flexibility exercises performed in the evening can decrease morning stiffness (Byers, 1985).

Resistance Exercises

Resistance against gravity, water, or another part of the body is often sufficient muscle training in inflammatory arthritis when significant weakness and atrophy are present. As strength is gained, however, it may be possible to add weights and load the muscle beyond gravitational forces to continue to build strength. Strength training is particularly important for older adults with rheumatoid arthritis as it is the only kind of exercise than can reverse the muscle wasting caused by catabolic cytokinemia (release of high levels of cytokines that elevate metabolic rates and cause wasting of skeletal muscle), which is part of the disease process (Ettinger et al., 1998).

BARRIERS TO EXERCISE

Despite the known benefits of exercise and the fact that there is little risk of damage to joints from regular moderate-intensity exercise in individuals with arthritis, it is particularly challenging to motivate these individuals to initiate and/or adhere to a regular exercise program (Ettinger et al., 1997; Sullivan, Allegrante, Peterson, Kovar, & MacKenzie, 1998). To maximize adherence to exercise programs it is useful to consider the many factors that are known to influence motivation with regard to exercise in older adults. The theory of self-efficacy has been useful in identifying those factors. This theory suggests that the stronger the individual's efficacy expectations (self-efficacy and outcome expectations), the more likely he or she will initiate and persist with a given activity. Outcome expectations are the beliefs that there will be a specific outcome following a behavior. Self-efficacy expectations are the individuals' beliefs in their capabilities to perform a certain activity.

Both self-efficacy and outcome expectations play an influential role in the adoption and maintenance of exercise behavior in older adults (Fitzgerald, Singleton, Neale, Prasad, & Hess, 1994; Lachman, et al., 1997; McAuley, 1993; McAuley, Shaffer & Rudolph, 1995; Resnick, 1998; Sharpe & McConnell, 1992). Older adults may have high self-efficacy expectations for exercise, but if they do not believe the exercise will improve health, strength, or function, or if they believe that exercise will make the arthritis worse, then it is unlikely that they will adhere to a regular exercise program. Efficacy expectations are dynamic and are based on four sources of information: (1) performance accomplishment, or successfully performing the activity; (2) verbal persuasion, or being told you are capable of performing the activity; (3) role models, or seeing like individuals perform a specific activity; and (4) physiological or affective states such as pain, fatigue, or anxiety associated with a given activity.

Using this theoretical framework, and studies specifically exploring the factors that influence exercise behavior in older adults (Conn, 1998; Resnick, 1998; Resnick, Palmer, Jenkins & Spellbring, 2000; Resnick & Spellbring, 2000; Sharon, Hennessy, Brandon & Boyette, 1997), a seven step approach (Resnick, 1999) was developed to help motivate older adults to exercise. The seven step approach addresses all of the commonly identified barriers described by older adults as decreasing their adherence to a regular exercise program.

The Seven Step Approach

Step I: Education

Education about the benefits of exercise is an essential first step to helping older adults start an exercise program. This is particularly true for older adults with arthritis as many of these individuals continue to believe that simply resting joints and avoiding activity is the best way to manage their arthritis. Education about exercise, specifically what type and amount of exercise is needed and what benefits can be expected from regular exercise, helps to strengthen self-efficacy and outcome expectations related to exercise. Friedrich, Gittler, Halbertadt, Cermak, and Heiller(1998) used extensive counseling and information strategies that emphasized the importance of regular and consistent exercise for older adults with arthritis, and Resnick (2001) used one-on-one teaching by reviewing a specially developed exercise booklet for older adults that addresses the benefits and barriers to regular exercise. Appendix B (p. 154) provides an overview of the information that should be included in any teaching program. To facilitate learning, the information should be given in multiple formats: an interactive lecture, a written handout, or a videotape. The information must be repeated and reinforced both informally (one-on-one with older adults), and formally in teaching programs.

Older adults, particularly those who have been sedentary, need additional education regarding normal responses to exercise and how to recognize the warning signs of excessive exercise (Table 9.4). It is important that older adults understand the difference between *normal* responses to exercise and those that are abnormal so that they do not use the normal responses to exercise as an excuse to stop exercising.

Step II. Exercise Pre-screening

From a motivational perspective, screening is important to assure individuals that they can succeed in the exercise program initiated. Moreover, successfully passing a screening evaluation for exercise reinforces to exercisers that they are capable of exercising regularly, and decreases the barrier that fear of dying or experiencing a cardiac event during exercise can pose (Resnick & Spellbring, 2000).

TABLE 9.4 Normal Responses to Exercise and Warning Signs of Excessive Exercise

Normal Response to Exercise	Warning Signs of Excessive Exercise
Increased heart rate and breathing mild perspiration an increased awareness of one's heartbeat mild muscle aches	severe dyspnea wheezing coughing chest pain or discomfort excessive perspiration dizziness prolonged fatigue lasting at least half an hour after exercise joint stress that includes joint pain during or for more than 1 to 2 hours after exercise, joint swelling, fatigue, or weakness

Step III. Setting Goals

Self-monitoring and goal setting can be used to recognize, prompt, and reward exercise behavior (King, Rejeski & Buchner, 1998). Goals should be clear, specific, and attainable, and must realistically fit into the individual's daily schedule. Goals should explicitly state the type and amount of effort needed to attain them, and ideally should be set to be moderately difficult. Relatively easy goals are not challenging enough to arouse much interest or effort, and goals set well beyond one's reach can be demotivating by undermining the individual's self-efficacy expectations. Goals set at the beginning of the program should focus on the amount of time the individual is expected to participate in exercise, rather than the extent of exertion. This lessens the pressure the individual might feel to perform a more challenging task, which might only decrease motivation if the person is unable to do it.

Examples of initial exercise goals are walking three times a week for 20 minutes at one's own pace, and doing a series of resistive exercise for 20 to 30 minutes at least twice a week. Examples of long term goals include experiencing less knee pain, taking less medication, being able to walk faster, losing weight, walking further before becoming short of breath, walking without an assistive device, or taking a vacation that requires a certain level of physical activity. Ideally, goals should be reviewed weekly so that positive reinforcement of goal attainment can be given, and goals can be revised as appropriate.

Step IV: Exposure to Exercise

Actual performance of the activity of interest can strengthen efficacy expectations in adults and thereby improve motivation and behavior (McAuley et al., 1995; Resnick, 1998; 2000). Sometimes older adults are not exercising simply because they do not know what to do, and may worry about making symptoms worse. These individuals may not have had prior experience with regular exercise and may be unable to establish an exercise program independently. Therefore it is very helpful to set some clear guidelines about how to exercise, and write out exactly what should be done. Appendix A provides a useful list of resources that give details of exercise programs. The individual should have some general guidelines as well, such as those recommended by the American College of Sports Medicine (Table 9.5).

Even with this information provided, motivating older adults with arthritis to participate in their first exercise session is often difficult. Table 9.6 reviews the common barriers older adults with arthritis

TABLE 9.5 Guidelines for Exercise Programs for Older Adults with Arthritis

Guideline	Rationale for Guideline
Begin slow and progress gradually	Progress gradually with regard to intensity, complexity, and duration.
	This will prevent exacerbation of the arthritis pain or functional impairment.
	Exercise daily when pain and stiffness are minimal (evenings).
Avoid rapid or repetitive movements of affects joints	Protect the joints during exercise and avoid activities that require rapid repetitions of a movement or those that are highly percussive.
	Avoid fast walking, which increases joint stress.
	Control pronation and shock absorption for the feet by choosing appropriate shoes or using orthotics.
Adapt physical activity to the needs of the individual	Joints that are restricted with regard to range of motion by pain, stiffness, swelling, or bone changes may require additional care to prevent injury.
	Use appropriate joint protection during exercise.

TABLE 9.6 Ways to Address Barriers to Exercise

Barrier	Suggested Ways to Overcome the Barrier
Not enough time	Incorporate activity into your daily life: park as far as possible from your destination; walk to work; walk up the stairs; spend 20 minutes walking after work and skip a TV show.
Exercise causes pain	Use appropriate pain relieving medications such as Tylenol, or ice joints prior to exercise. Remember also that exercise is the best way to decrease pain from osteoarthritis or osteoporosis.
Exercise is boring	Do an activity you enjoy. Listen to a book on tape, a radio, or music. Exercise with a friend and walk and talk.
Exercise is too tiring	Take a rest prior to exercising. Also remember that exercise will actually increase your energy level.
I am afraid of falling	Choose a safe, well-lit, flat area to walk and remember that exercise is the best way to strengthen muscles, improve balance, and decrease the risk of falling.
I am afraid of getting hurt	Walking and swimming are very safe exercises that will not stress joints or muscles.
I am too old to exercise	You will benefit from regular exercise no matter what age you are. You can improve your strength, balance, and cardiovascular health, as well as overall mood and well-being by exercising when you are older.
I am too fat to exercise	Being overweight is a good reason to exercise. It is safe as long as you follow the right guidelines and begin with a low to moderate-intensity activity such as walking.
There is no place to exercise	Choose an activity you can do in a convenient place; walk outside if it is safe or in the hallways of an apartment building. Another option is to pick a stair and do some stair walking and stepping.
I don't see any reason to exercise; I don't want to live forever!	Exercise may not dramatically increase the length of your life but it will increase the quality by helping you stay as healthy and independent as possible.

TABLE 9.7 Interventions to Decrease Unpleasant Sensations Associated with Exercise

Problem	Intervention
Pain	Have participant take pain medication one half hour prior to exercise. If not effective, in conjunction with the primary care provider, alter current medication regime. Implement use of ice/heat as appropriate prior to and following exercise. Educate/encourage that exercise will help reduce pain. Implement relaxation techniques as appropriate. Implement guided imagery as appropriate.
Fear	Educate/encourage that exercise will prevent future falls. Assure individuals that they will not be asked to do exercises they are not capable of performing safely. Educate/encourage that exercise will not damage arthritic joints but rather will strengthen them. Encourage verbalization of fears. Implement relaxation techniques as appropriate. Implement guided imagery as appropriate. Implement distraction techniques. Use hip protectors.
Fatigue	Stress the importance of exercise to combat fatigue and improve sleep. Encourage one half hour rest period prior to exercise activity. In conjunction with the primary care provider evaluate for other causes of fatigue including anemia, electrolyte imbalance, drug side effects, infection, dehydration, or altered nutritional status. Educate regarding sleep patterns for older adults and ways to naturally facilitate sleep.

report as reasons that prevent them from initiating an exercise program. Reviewing these and providing the individual with a reasonable solution to each barrier will decrease the influence of these barriers and help the individual initiate the first exercise session. It is particularly important to address the unpleasant sensations associated with exercise such as pain, fear of hurting the joint, fear of falling or getting hurt, or fatigue, and to provide the individual with ways to decrease these sensations (Table 9.7). Once the first exercise session is completed, individuals should be reminded of their success with that exercise session, and encouraged to continue.

Step V: Exposure to Role Models

Exposure to role models, or seeing similar individuals successfully perform an activity, can help older adults believe that they too are capable of performing that activity (Bandura, 1997; Chogahara, 1999; Resnick, 1998). Introducing your patient to an older adult with arthritis who exercises regularly and can describe the benefits of this behavior can be a great source of encouragement and motivation. Health care providers should also be role models and share their own exercise experiences, how they overcome barriers to exercise, and their exercise successes.

Step VI: Verbal Encouragement

Verbal encouragement from a trusted, credible source has been used alone, and with performance behavior, to strengthen efficacy expectations related to exercise (Courneya & McAuley, 1995; Resnick, 1996, 1998). Verbal encouragement to begin an exercise program should be given to patients not only by their primary health care provider, but ideally from all of those individuals they interact with in the health care delivery system. Older adults should be repeatedly assured that they are capable of participating in a regular exercise program. Once exercise activities are initiated, verbal encouragement should be given to continue to exercise, with a major emphasis placed on both the mental and physical health benefits of regular exercise.

Step VII: Verbal Reinforcement/Rewards

Rewards have been identified as an important aspect of motivation to exercise. Unfortunately it is particularly difficult to identify appropriate rewards for older adults. Jette et al. (1998) used tangible rewards, (colored magnets) when older adults in a home-based exercise program demonstrated increased exercise intensity. Older adults have reported that verbal reinforcement, kindness, and caring from their health care providers were perceived as rewards for their participation in exercise activities (Resnick, 1996,1998). Exercisers should be praised and applauded for their efforts and reminded of the positive health benefits they receive from exercising regularly. Genuine excitement by the health care provider should be demonstrated in response to evidence of exercise activities or the patient's achievement of a goal.

More concrete rewards or benefits of exercise for older adults with arthritis are changes in joint range of motion and strength, and decreased weight. The nurse, and/or the patient can keep a monthly record of markers such as range of motion, strength and/or weight, compile this information, and thereby continually evaluate progress. These important physical benefits of adhering to an exercise program are a great way to motivate your exercisers to "keep up the good work."

USE OF PHYSICAL AND OCCUPATIONAL THERAPY

Physical and occupational therapy play central roles in the management of individuals with arthritis because of the commonly associated functional limitations. The physical therapist assesses muscle strength, joint stability, and mobility, and can help prescribe specific exercise programs and pain management techniques. For example, the physical therapist can individually establish an exercise program for the older adult with arthritis. This program may focus on improving joint range of motion and periarticular muscle strength, and/ or teaching these individuals the use of assistive devices such as canes, crutches or walkers that will improve ambulation, protect the joints, and allow for aerobic exercise activity.

Older adults with arthritis commonly present with quadriceps weakness. This weakness is due to disuse atrophy, which develops because of unloading of the painful extremity. Physical therapy can have a beneficial effect on quadricep strengthening in these individuals. Sensory dysfunction, reflected by a decrease in proprioception, is also common in older adults with arthritis. Physical therapy can help to improve knee joint position sense, quadriceps strength, and performance in activities of daily living.

Use of Assistive Devices

The appropriate and safe use of assistive devices is also an important component of physical therapy for older adults with arthritis. The proper use of a cane (i.e., in the hand contralateral to the affected knee) reduces loading forces on the joint and is associated with a decrease in pain and improvement of function. In addition, older adults may benefit from wedged insoles to correct abnormal biomechanics due to changes in the knee joint. Another useful maneuver that can be done best under the guidance of a physical therapist, particularly in individuals who have patellofemoral compartment involvement, is medial taping of the patella (Cushnaghan, McCarthy, & Dieppe, 1994).

Some older adults with arthritis may benefit from a referral to a physical therapist or exercise specialist to help them develop an exercise program. The therapists can carefully assess joint motion, muscle strength and endurance, and performance of activities of daily living. The exercise program can then be individualized to meet the specific needs of that individual, and can include electrophysical agents to supplement exercise including laser, interferential ultrasound, and local heat treatment. Adherence to this program can be helped using the techniques described above. Group physical therapy programs have also been found to be effective in decreasing knee pain and improving function. The group programs focus on exercise using stationary bicycles, weights, and machines allowing for both eccentric (muscle is lengthened) and concentric (muscle is shortened) lower limb strengthening, stairs and a stepper machine.

NON-PHARMACOLOGICAL PAIN MANAGEMENT

Pain management is another area in which physical therapists can improve the care provided for older adults with arthritis. Transcutaneous nerve stimulation (TENS), electroacupuncture, and ice massage have all been shown to be effective pain management techniques. In addition, physical therapists can evaluate the patient for the use of bracing and corrective footwear. Shock-absorbing footwear reduces the damaging impact of loading, heel wedging reduces the later thrust on the knee, support sleeves increase proprioception and reduce overall feelings of instability, dynamic bracing controls lateral instability, and taping of the knee allows repositioning of the patella (Felson et al., 2000).

The occupational therapist can be instrumental in directing individuals in proper joint protection, modification of daily tasks, and energy conservation, including the use of splints and other assistive devices to help improve range of motion and joint function.

SUMMARY

Although many older adults continue to believe they should rest an arthritic joint, it has repeatedly been demonstrated that regular exercise will improve joint function, decrease pain, and improve balance. The specific goals of exercise in arthritis are to prevent deconditioning of the muscles and keep the joints stable, to improve joint flexibility, and to enhance aerobic fitness, while maintaining good joint protection. Muscles that do not get used regularly because of pain will atrophy. A comprehensive exercise program should, therefore, include stretching exercises, followed by a range-of-motion program for the joint, muscle strengthening, and aerobic exercise. Muscle strengthening, or resistance training is not recommended for a severely inflamed joint. However, once the acute episode resolves, muscle strengthening should be resumed to prevent muscle atrophy around inflamed joints.

Despite the known benefits of exercise it is challenging to motivate older adults with arthritis to initiate and engage in a regular exercise program. The Seven Step Approach provides a practical framework to help overcome the barriers to exercise and improve exercise activity in these individuals.

REFERENCES

Arthritis: A leading cause of disability in the United States. (2000). *National Academy on An Aging Society, 5,* 1–6.

Bandura A. (1997). *Self-efficacy: The exercise of control.* New York: W. H. Freeman.

Borg, G. (1982). Psychosocial bases of perceived exertion. *Medicine Science Sports and Exercise, 472,* 194–381.

Bostrom, C., Harms-Ringdahl, K., Karreskog, H., & Nordemar, R. (1998). Effects of static and dynamic shoulder rotator exercises in women with rheumatoid arthritis: A randomized comparison of impairment, disability, handicap, and health. *Scandinavian Journal of Rheumatology 27,* 281–290.

Byers, P. (1985). Effects of exercise on morning stiffness and mobility in patients with rheumatoid arthritis. *Research in Nursing and Health, 8,* 275–280.

Cushnaghan, J., McCarthy, C., & Dieppe, P. (1994). Taping the patella medially: A new treatment for osteoarthritis of the knee joint. *British Medical Journal, 308,* 752–53.

Chogahara, M. (1999). A multidimensional scale for assessing positive and negative social influences on physical activity in older adults. *Journal of Gerontology: Social Science, 54B,* S356–368.

Conn, V. (1998). Older adults and exercise. *Nursing Research, 47,* 180–189.

Courneya, K. S., & McAuley, E. (1995). Cognitive mediators of the social influence-exercise adherence relationship: A test of the theory of planned behavior. *Journal of Behavioral Medicine, 18*(5), 499–515.

Deyle G. D., Henderson, N. E., Matekel R. L., Ryder, M. G., Garber, M. B., & Allison S. C. (2000). Effectiveness of manual physical therapy and exercise in osteoarthritis of the knee: A randomized controlled trial. *Annals of Internal Medicine, 132,* 173–181.

Ettinger, W. H., Fried, L. P., Harris, T., Schemanski, L., Schultz, R., & Robbins, J. (1994). Self reported causes of physical disability in older people: The Cardiovascular Health Study. *Journal of the American Geriatrics Society, 42,* 1035–1044.

Ettinger, S. H., Burns, R., Messier, S. P., Applegate, W., Rejeski, W. J., Morgan, T., Shumaker, S., Berry, M. J., O'Toole, M., Monu, J., & Craven, T. (1997). A randomized trial comparing aerobic exercise and resistance exercise with a health education program in older adults with knee osteoarthritis. *Journal of American Medical Association, 277,* 25–31.

Ettinger, W. H., Jr. (1994). Physical activity, arthritis, and disability in older people. *Musculoskeletal Connective Tissue Disorders, 14,* 633–640.

Felson, D., Lawrence, R., Hochberg, M., McAlindon, T., Dicppe, P., Minor, M., et al., (2000). Osteoarthritis: New insights, Part 2: Treatment Approaches. *Annals of Internal Medicine, 133*(9), 726-737.

Fitzgerald, J., Singleton, S., Neale, A., Prasad, A., & Hess, J. (1994). Activity levels, fitness status, exercise knowledge, and exercise beliefs among healthy, older African American and white women. *Journal of Aging and Health, 6,* 296–313.

Fransen, Crosbie, & Edmonds, J. (2001). Physical therapy is effective for patients with osteoarthritis of the knee: a randomized controlled clinical trial. *The Journal of Rheumatology, 28,* 156–164.

Friedrich, M., Gittler, G., Halberstadt, Y., Cermak, T., & Heiller, I. (1998). Combined exercise and motivation program: Effect on the compliance and level of disability of patients with chronic low back pain: a randomized controlled trial. *Archives of Physical Medicine and Rehabilitation 79,* 475–489.

Jette, A., Lachman, M., Giorgetti, M., Assmann, S., Harris, B., Levensen, C., Wernick, M., & Krebs, D. (1998). Effectiveness of home-based resistance training with disabled older persons. *The Gerontologist, 38,* 412–422.

Hurley, M. V. & Scott, D. L. (1998). Improvements in quadriceps sensorimotor function and disability of patients with knee osteoarthritis following a clinically practical exercise regime. *British Journal of Rheumatology, 37,* 1181–1187.

King, A., Rejeski, J., & Buchner, D. (1998). Physical activity interventions targeting older adults: A critical review. *American Journal of Preventive Medicine, 15,* 316–333.

Lachman M, Jette A, Tennstedt S, Howland J, Harris B. & Peterson E. (1997). A cognitive-behavioral model for promoting regular physical activity in older adults. *Psychology, Health & Medicine, 2,* 251–261.

Lane, N. E., & Buckwalter, J. A. (1993). Exercise: A cause of osteoarthritis? *Rheumatic Disease Clinics of North America, 19*(3), 617–33

Mangione, K. K., McCully, K., Gloviak, A., Lefebvre, I., Hofmann, M., & Craik, R. (1999). The effects of high-intensity and low-intensity cycle ergometry in older adults with knee osteoarthritis. *Journal of Gerontology, A54,* M184–M190.

Maurer, B. T., Stern, A. G., Kinossian, B., Cook, K. D., & Schumacher, H. R., Jr. (1999).Osteoarthritis of the knee: Isokinetic quadriceps exercise versus an educational intervention. *Archives of Physical Medicine and Rehabilitation, 80,* 293–1299.

Messier, S. P., Thompson, C. D., & Ettinger, W. H., Jr. (1997). Effects of long term aerobic or weight training regimens on gait in an older, osteoarthritis population. *Journal of Applied Biomechanics, 13,* 205–225.

McAuley, E. (1993). Self-efficacy and the maintenance of exercise participation in older adults. *Journal of Behavioral Medicine, 16,* 103–113.

McAuley, E., Shaffer, K., & Rudolph, D. (1995). Effective response to acute exercise in elderly impaired males: The moderating effects of self-efficacy and age. *International Journal of Aging and Human Development, 41,* 13–27.

Messier, S. P., Royer, T. D., Craven, T. E., O'Toole, M. L., Burns, R., & Ettinger, W. H. (2000). Long-term exercise and its effect on balance in older osteoarthritic adults: Results from the fitness, arthreitis seniors trial (FAST). *Journal of the American Geriatrics Society, 48,* 131–138.

National Institute of Arthritis and Musculoskeletal and Skin Disease, National Institutes of Health. (1998). *Arthritis prevalence rising as baby boomers grow older.* Available at: *http://www.nih.gov./niams*

O'Reilly, S. C., Muir, K. R., & Doherty, M. (1999). Effectiveness of home exercise on pain and disability from osteoarthritis of the knee: A randomized controlled trial. *Annals of Rheumatological Disease, 58,* 15–19.

Resnick, B. (1994). The wheel that moves. *Rehabilitation Nursing, 19*(4), 18.

Resnick, B. (1996). Motivation in geriatric rehabilitation. *Image 28*, 41–47.

Resnick, B. (1998). Self-efficacy in geriatric rehabilitation. *Journal of Gerontological Nursing, 24*, 34–44.

Resnick, B. (1999, March 8). Exercise for the Older Adult: The seven step approach to wellness. *Advance for Nurses, 20.*

Resnick, B. (2000). Functional performance and exercise of older adults in long term care. *Journal of Gerontological Nursing, 26*(3), 7–16.

Resnick B. (2001). Testing a model of exercise behavior in older adults. *Reasearch in Nursing Health, 24*(2), 83-92.

Resnick, B., Palmer, M. H., Jenkins, L., & Spellbring, A. M. (2000). Efficacy expectations and exercise behavior in older adults: A path analysis. *Journal of Advanced Nursing, 32*(1), 13–26.

Resnick, B., & Spellbring, A. M. (2000). Understanding what motivates older adults to exercise. *Journal of Gerontologic Nursing, 26*(3), 34–42.

Sharon, B., Hennessy, C., Brandon, J., & Boyette, L. (1997). Older adults' experiences of a strength training program. *The Journal of Nutrition, Health & Aging, 1*, 103–108.

Sharpe, P., & McConnell, C. (1992). Exercise beliefs and behaviors among older employees: A health promotion trial. *The Gerontologist, 32*, 444–449.

Slemenda, C., Brandt, K., Heilman, D., Mazzuca, S., Braunstein, E., & Katz, B. (1997). Quadriceps weakness and osteoarthritis of the knee. *Annals of Internal Medicine, 127*, 97–104).

Spencer, A. C., Kinne, S., Belza, B. L., Ramsey, S., & Patrick, D. L. (1998). Recruiting adults with osteoarthritis into an aquatic exercise class: Strategies for a statewide intervention. *Arthritis Care Research, 11*, 455–462.

Sullivan, T., Allegrante, J. P., Peterson, M. G., Kovar, P. A., & MacKenzie, C. R. (1998). One-year follow-up of patients with osteoarthritis of the knee who participated in a program of supervised fitness walking and supportive patient education. *Arthritis Care Research, 11*(4), 228–233.

Van Baar, M. E., Dekker, J., Oostendorp, R. A., Bijl, D., Voorn, T. B., Lemmens, J. A., & Bijlsma, J. W. (1998). The effectiveness of exercise therapy in patients with osteoarthritis of the hip or knee: A randomized clinical trial. *Journal of Rheumatology, 25*, 2431–2439.

Van den Ende, C. H., Vliet Vlieland, T. P., Munneke, M., & Hazes, J. M. (1998). Dynamic exercise therapy in rheumatoid arthritis: A systematic review. *British Journal of Rheumatology, 37*(6), 677–687.

APPENDIX A: Resources for Developed Exercise Programs for Older Adults

1. *Exercise: A Guide from the National Institute on Aging.* Publication No. NIH 99–4258. Internet address: *http://www.nih.gov/nia*
2. *Living with Exercise: Improving Your Health Through Moderate Physical Activity,* Steven N. Blair, P.E.D., American Health Publishing Company, Dallas, TX, 1991
3. *Activating Ideas: Promoting Physical /Activity Among Older Adults,* AARP, 601 E. Street N.W., Washington, DC 20049, Phone (202) 434–2230
4. *The Exercise Plus Program.* Barbara Resnick, National Institute on Aging Grant No. RO1 AG17082–01. Contact bresnick@umaryland.edu

APPENDIX B: Program for Teaching Older Adults About Exercise

I. Benefits of Exercise (stretching, resistive and aerobic activity]
   • improve strength, balance, and maximum aerobic capacity, and decrease joint stress
   • prevent diseases/disability
   • decrease pain
   • decrease the risk of falling or getting hurt
   • improve sleep
   • enhances mood and general well-being
II. Specific Physical Changes that Result from Regular Exercise
   • increase in blood flow to the muscle
   • increased oxygen consumption/ventilation
   • increased consumption of free fatty acids
   • increase in cardiac output, decrease in heart rate and blood pressure
   • decrease in peripheral vascular resistance
   • increase in maximum aerobic capacity (VO_2 Max)
   • improved bone density
   • increase in brain serotonin synthesis
III. Appropriate Goals to Achieve Benefits of Exercise
   • include daily stretching, resistive exercise at least 2 x per week, and aerobic activity at least 3 x per week.
   • begin at low levels and gradually increase to 60 to 80% of maximal heart rate (MHR). To calculate 70% of MHR the formula 220–age x .70 is used.
IV. Recognition of the Warning Signs of Excessive Exercise
   • These signs include severe dyspnea, wheezing, coughing, chest discomfort, excessive perspiration, syncope, prolonged fatigue (lasting greater than one half hour after exercise), or local muscle or joint discomfort.
V. Beating the Barriers to Exercise
   • Choose an activity you find pleasurable
   • Choose a convenient, economical activity
   • Set realistic goals
   • Structure your exercise so it is set in your schedule
   • Remember that exercise won't make you more tired-it cures fatigue
   • Remember that exercise won't hurt arthritis-it helps reduce pain
   • Remember that you are never too old to exercise or to benefit from exercise

10
Patient Teaching Tools and Self-Help Techniques: Focus on Cultural Diversity

Ann Mabe Newman

The National Arthritis Plan (Center for Disease Control and Prevention, 1999) calls on health care providers to develop strategies to engage people with arthritis who do not participate in self-management programs. Special considerations for the older adult with arthritis need to be given attention. Statistics alone demand that providers design programs with the older adult in mind because by 2030, 22% of the population will be older than 65. The demographic characteristics of older adults with arthritis have been presented in chapter 1, and certainly, the specific self-help techniques for the city dweller will differ from those used with the rural dweller. However, the principles of self-help presented here remain the same. The purpose of this chapter is to describe the principles of some of the self-help techniques and many teaching tools available to help older adults with arthritis to live more comfortably. After an example of how these self-help principles were used in a program to help older African-American adults with arthritis, nursing and medical implications will be presented.

DEFINITIONS AND DESCRIPTION

Self-help/self-management is a term that is widely interpreted and a formal definition may be helpful. Self-help/self-management is defined as being responsible for decision-making related to your own health. Monitoring one's own health not only includes making informed decisions about when to use health care providers and practicing appropriate health behaviors, it also includes using family, friends, and community resources when appropriate. Self-help/self-management uses a problem-solving approach to make decisions (Lorig, 1996). This term is presented in the context of the more widely used term *patient education*, which is commonly defined as any set of planned educational activities intended to improve a patient's health behaviors. At this time, reimbursement policies rarely allow sufficient time for patient education, including a demonstration of new skills. Good patient education programs have always focused on more than disease management. Current cost effectiveness practices have necessitated a look at other ways of accomplishing these goals.

Teaching people to self-manage a disease such as arthritis, is fast becoming the norm. The self-management model has at least three distinguishing features as described by Lorig (1996): (1) dealing with the consequences of the disease, not just the physiological disease; (2) being concerned with problem solving, decision making, and patient confidence, rather than merely with prescription and adherence; and (3) placing patients and health professionals in partnership relationships. After medical/nursing management of the disease, the patient is primarily responsible for the day-to-day management of the illness. Communication is the key to full partnership between the patient and the health professional.

ARTHRITIS SELF-MANAGEMENT

Arthritis self-help intervention programs have become an important part of ameliorating the effects of living with arthritis. These programs have demonstrated their effectiveness in reducing the burden of illness, improving health-related quality of life, and reducing health care costs (Lorig, Mazonson, & Holman (1993). The Arthritis Self-Help Course (ASHC), which is endorsed by the Arthritis Foundation

(Arthritis Foundation, 1997), is an example of a successful self-help program. The goals of the Arthritis Self-Help Course are to (1) inform participants about basic aspects of arthritis and joint anatomy; (2) teach principles of exercise and provide an opportunity to practice stretching and strengthening exercises; (3) teach principles of joint protection and energy conservation and provide an opportunity to share ideas about improving one's functional ability; (4) teach the appropriate utilization of arthritis medications; (5) encourage informed decisions about the use of special diets and nontraditional forms of treatment; (6) encourage participants to take an active role in arthritis management and make appropriate use of arthritis care providers; (7) encourage sharing of experiences and group problem solving; (8) and provide an opportunity for learning and practicing stress management and other self-help behaviors designed to decrease stress, pain, and depression (Lorig, 1997).

The ASHC is a six–week, group education, community-based program in which participants learn principles of self-management, receive information on medications and nutrition, and learn about the relationship between pain and depression. They participate in problem solving, and practice communication skills, relaxation techniques, and exercise. Participants are given homework assignments to complete between sessions. Leaders complete a two-day training session. Lay people or professionals can teach the course. The course content emphasizes experiential activities to assist persons with arthritis to feel more confident in self-managing their arthritis. The content and process of the ASHC are standardized as outlined in the ASHC Leader's Manual (Lorig, 1997). For two to two and a half hours per week, over six consecutive weeks, participants engage in experiential learning covering specific content in each session. The course covers the following topics: arthritis/joint anatomy, self-help principles, pain control, exercise, relaxation, dealing with depression, communicating with your caregiver; nutrition, nontraditional treatment, and self-care and self-efficacy.

The ASHC uses skills mastery, modeling, reinterpreting symptoms and changing beliefs, and contracts to enhance self-care. It is based on research findings indicating that such a program is effective in enhancing self-efficacy, or confidence in one's ability to accomplish a specific behavior. Several studies indicate a relationship between increased self-efficacy and increased adaptation to arthritis with improvements in health status, including the perception of decreased pain and increased perceived ability to manage symptoms (Lorig & Gonzalez, 1992; Lorig, Mazonson, & Holman, 1989; Newman, 1993). In addition to self-efficacy, research findings have revealed that various individual mediating variables may be important in how the program works to improve health status and decrease perceived pain, although how they interact is not clear (Lorig, Chastain, Ung, Shoor & Holman, 1989).

RESEARCH WITH AFRICAN AMERICANS WITH ARTHRITIS

Although elderly Caucasians and African Americans have similar rates of arthritis, greater rates of activity limitations are found among African Americans. Arthritis is the third most common health problem among African Americans and the leading cause of activity limitations (U.S. Department of Health and Human Services, 1998). Adapting to living with the consequences of arthritis is a serious health problem, particularly for minorities, because some of the obstacles that face people experiencing health care problems fall disproportionately on older racial and ethnic minority populations within our society (U.S. Department of Health and Human Services, 1996). Receiving care that is perceived as racially and ethnically relevant is an important factor in overcoming the obstacles. African American elders continue to have less health insurance than their Caucasian counterparts; thus, African-American elders are less likely to be able to afford health care (Dennis & Neese, 2000).

Because little research as been conducted with African Americans with arthritis, the following example of using the ASHC in an African American community is presented. In the pilot study by Stephenson, Yee, and Lisse (1997) with 26 older African Americans with arthritis, the authors concluded that "the findings from this pilot suggest that the Arthritis Self-Help Course program may be an appropriate and effective cognitive-behavioral intervention for African Americans with arthritis" (p. 85).

Newman (2001) conducted a follow-up research study to better understand the effects of arthritis self-help intervention in older African Americans who lack resources to seek health care. The specific aim was to answer the questions: (1) What is the effect of the Arthritis Self-Help Course (ASHC) on arthritis self-efficacy in older African Americans? (2) What is the relationship of arthritis self-efficacy to perceived social support and spiritual health?

One hundred and fifty African Americans, with arthritis, over age 55, participated in the study. Participants were predominately older (mean age of 65), retired, with a mean educational level of 3.6 years, African-American women living in public housing in a large southeastern city. A pretest-posttest design was used to investigate differences in self-efficacy in ASHC participants and a control group. The instruments administered were a demographic data sheet, the Arthritis Self-Efficacy Scales (ASES) (Lorig, Chastain, Ung, Shoor, & Holman, 1989), the Personal Resource Questionnaire (PRQ85), (Weinert, 1987), the Spiritual Well-Being Scale (SWB) (Ellison, 1983) and a Visual Analogue Scale for pain (VAS). Subjects were assigned to control or treatment groups and the treatment groups. The control groups were offered the opportunity to take the course after the study period.

As hypothesized, participants in the ASHC increased their self-efficacy for management of pain and other symptoms (p<.05). Associations between the scores on the Visual Analogue Scale and the scores on the Arthritis Self-Efficacy Scales were as expected: negatively correlated and statistically significant, that is, the higher the self-efficacy for pain and other symptom management, the lower the perceived pain. Newman (2001) concluded that people with arthritis who received the intervention of the Arthritis Self-Help Course had higher self-efficacy scores than people in the control group. However, the tools used to measure the study variables need to be adapted for use in a population of African-American elders with low reading comprehension.

Restricted space allows for only a few of the rich anecdotal stories encountered during the conduct of this research. They are cited as evidence of the flexibility of the ASHC as a prototype for nursing interventions to help people with arthritis and other chronic diseases feel more confident in managing their illnesses. Throughout the program, participants are asked to share techniques that help them to manage their arthritis. They reported, as did an earlier study by Bill-Harvey, Rippey, Abeles, & Pfeiffer (1989), that prayer, canes, and heat were most efficacious for them. "I pray and read my Bible, and

Jesus gives me strength to face another day," reported one participant.

While all of the material as outlined must be covered, the leader
can use discussion times to build trust and give participants the
notion that they can speak freely without fearing they will be told
that what they are doing won't help. Unless the leader has evidence
that the practice is harmful, it should not be condemned.

One morning I arrived at a church where I was to teach an arthritis self-help course. I had missed my turn off the freeway, I was late,
the rain was pouring down, and I was very wet. To my surprise, on
the steps stood an 80–year old woman, alone, with her umbrella
poised over her gray head, and a radiant smile on her face. "How
did you get here," I asked. " I took the bus and transferred twice,"
she replied. "How long have you been here?" I continued. "Oh,
about an hour, I didn't want to be late," she responded. She seemed
genuinely puzzled when I told her she probably should be teaching
the class! So be prepared-for some older adults with arthritis, self-
help is a state of mind.

With its emphasis on self-management and increasing self-efficacy, programs like the ASHC can be prototypes developed to incorporate coping methods that are preferred by other ethnic groups while
maintaining the integrity of the research-based educational intervention. *The Self-Help Course Manual* (Lorig, 1997) and *The Arthritis Helpbook* (Lorig & Fries, 1995) are available from the Arthritis Foundation
in all 50 states. These sources provide information on the making or
ordering of relaxation tapes, as well as a variety of inexpensive items
clients can make. Two suggestions from African American elders
participating in the research were cutting the legs off discarded panty
hose and using the stretchable tops to encourage gentle arm and
shoulder stretching. These exercise bands are easier for seniors to
use than the more expensive latex exercise bands. Participants also
suggested using familiar gospel music tapes for exercise. Both in
previous studies (Dukski, & Newman, 1989; Newman,1993) and in
this study (Newman, 2001), simply teaching relaxation techniques
can decrease a client's perception of pain.

It has been estimated that by the year 2065, Caucasians will not be
the majority in this country (Francis, 1992). Therefore, it is imperative that nurses and other health care providers begin to look at
ways to provide culturally relevant care. Likewise, as the mean age

of the population increases, so too will the prevalence of this chronic illness. By the year 2030, 22% of the population will be over 65.

IMPORTANCE OF RACIAL AND ETHNIC ISSUES IN ARTHRITIS

Documentation that race and ethnic issues are of central importance to understanding of health and health behaviors was identified more than a decade ago (Cooper, 1991; Kumanyika & Golden, 1991). However, the health care system, including its practices and regimens, often fails to fully integrate the values and health-seeking behaviors of African Americans. Nursing and health care interventions for people with arthritis need to be based on information that is relevant to the population being served. The notion of enhancing adaptive belief systems when viewed from a nursing perspective has the potential for improving client care.

OTHER TEACHING TOOLS AND SELF-HELP TECHNIQUES

In addition to the Arthritis Self-Help Course, also known as the Arthritis Self-Management Course, there are other arthritis education courses that use the principles of self-help. An integrative review by Goeppinger and Lorig (1997) summarizes findings from community-based arthritis patient education studies conducted over the past 15 years. Goeppinger's (1995) community-based intervention for arthritis self-care, *Bone Up On Arthritis* (BUOA), has been successfully used with rural elders to increase performance of self-care behaviors and decrease feelings of helplessness. The reader is referred to these references for a more complete description of these programs. No shortage of materials exists for the nurse who wants to initiate arthritis self-help education with older adults. The Arthritis Foundation offers a wide variety of professional materials on the latest treatments and education on their web site at http://www.arthritis.org; www.arthritis.org

Helping older adults with arthritis take control of their disease begins with teaching them problem-solving techniques. In *The*

Arthritis Helpbook, Lorig and Fries (1995) describe the problem-solving method as consisting of eight basic steps, starting with identifying the source of difficulty. The next task is to pinpoint the source of the problem, followed by generating ideas that might solve it. Selecting the idea that the person thinks will be most likely to work and trying it out increases the likelihood of success. After assessing the results, the person can choose another idea from the list if the first one did not work. Utilizing resources is another important step in problem solving. And finally, accepting the fact that the problem may not be solved at this time helps to prevent frustration. As noted in the research example, the notion of self-efficacy, the belief that one is capable of controlling one's own behavior, has become an important part of the arthritis and gerontologic research literature (Kee, 2000). Increasingly, the concept is being used by practitioners as a basis for designing effective health education programs. So teaching older adults with arthritis to have confidence in their ability to problem solve is the crux of teaching self-management/self-help skills. There is literature on how to enhance self-efficacy, and design self-help patient education materials. It is not necessary to design your own. In addition to the Arthritis Foundation, other useful resources are *Teaching Patients with Low Literacy Skills* by Doak, Doak, and Root (1996), *Patient Education: A Practical Approach* by Lorig (1996) and *The Arthritis Helpbook* by Lorig and Fries (1995).

The following techniques are but a sample of the many self-management suggestions that have been found to be helpful in working with the older adult with arthritis. Most of them can be found and explained in greater detail in either *The Arthritis Helpbook* by Lorig and Fries (1995) or The Arthritis Foundation's *Tips for Good Living* (2000). Use the suggestions as a starting point with patients for generating their own ideas.

Self-Help Suggestions

1. Velcro is a good alternative to buttons, which can be hard to manage, or a buttonhook can be made with a wooden dowel and a large paper clip. For easier bathing, two washcloths can be sewn together to make a bath mitt.
2. Foam hair curlers can be used for a variety of tasks. Slipped over mascara or eyeliner brushes, eating utensils, or a tooth-

brush, the foam will increase the size of the handle. The foam curlers also make pens and pencils easier to grip. A pizza wheel makes cutting easier than a knife for many foods.

3. Many older adults are using computers for business and pleasure, so in addition to frequent breaks, the design of the computer work station needs careful attention. The use of a foot rest can be helpful. If the computer chair is not ergonomically designed, consider forearm supports or wrist rests and a small towel roll behind the lower back. The document holder needs to be the same height and distance as the person is from the screen. Laptop computers are convenient but they do not encourage the use of good body mechanics.

4. To keep joints warm during sleep, use an electric blanket or a sleeping bag placed between the sheets. Raised toilet seats are a must; for women it makes standing easier.

5. When shaking hands grasp the fingers or the wrist. First, to prevent squeezing the hand too hard. Most people with arthritis do not have the gnarled joints that would present a visual cue to others when shaking hands.

6. Raised flower beds allow the older adult with arthritis to continue this pleasurable activity of gardening. Enlist the aid of service organizations such as the Boy Scouts or Girl Scouts to elevate the flower beds.

7. The mantra for people with arthritis is "Wheels, wheels, wheels." Wheels help to avoid lifting and carrying groceries, tasks that often present a problem for those who live alone.

8. Helping to avoid fatigue can be accomplished in little ways. Duplicate most used items such as tape, scissors, tissues, and cleaners, and put them in the places where they are regularly used.

9. Encourage the use of positive self-talk. Role model this behavior by telling patients that most people do this privately and that talking out loud to one's self is very affirming. Encourage practice in front of a mirror.

10. Household hints, such as use of a wooden pizza paddle to help tuck in the sheets and blankets when making a bed, and putting a small rubber shower mat in the sink to keep pots and pans from moving while scrubbing them help to relieve stress on joints.

11. Canes give people the support and confidence they need and help prevent falls. A cane with a wide rubber tip can be individualized with fancy tape or a scarf. Use the cane in the hand opposite the bad side.
12. Distributing the weight of a load is an important item for people with arthritis. Carrying a shoulder bag or briefcase with a shoulder strap by placing the strap over the opposite shoulder can help to distribute the weight.
13. Allow older adults with arthritis a choice of music when exercising. If the music is familiar to them it may encourage them to exercise longer.
14. Teaching the older adult with arthritis how to get up from the floor is an important movement that should be practiced prior to an emergency need. This movement can be done by rolling on one side and then using the upper hand to push up enough to get the lower elbow from under the person. The person should gradually sit up, shift onto all fours, then crawl to the nearest chair and place the hands on the seat for support. This will allow putting weight on the hands before bringing the knee up until one foot is flat on floor. When both feet are flat on floor, the person can begin to straighten the legs, pausing while keeping the head down before standing up. After standing up straight, but before beginning to walk, the person should pause again.

NURSING IMPLICATIONS

The answer is in; arthritis self-help programs work. The question remains: Why aren't we doing it? The answer to this is not so easy. The most frequently cited reasons that arthritis self-help programs are not being practiced are time and money. However, leaders in the field maintain that with careful assessment of who could benefit from arthritis self-help education programs, the cost-effectiveness would become a moot point (Lorig, Mazonson, & Holman, 1993). The nurse-generalist working with older people with arthritis could provide the information necessary for making this determination through a careful assessment interview. The instruments used to assess the older adult's perceptions are easily administered and could be used by the nurse to implement a group teaching program based on the individual needs of each participant. The axiom in patient education, to start where the patient *is* and move him toward where he *needs* to be, is the same for the older adult with arthritis.

Bandura (1986) says that the self-efficacy skills necessary for successful self-management can be enhanced in four ways: skills mastery, modeling, reinterpretation of symptoms, and verbal persuasion. Nodhturft, et al. (2000) taught older adults with arthritis to use the self-efficacy techniques by having patients first formulate action plans. Many older people with arthritis are so overwhelmed from living with the daily effects of their disease that they have lost the ability to set and accomplish goals. They need to be taught how to break goals down into small achievable steps: what, when, how much, how often?

Bandura's notions of skills mastery can be taught by asking patients to try new behaviors every week and include time for discussion of problems. Modeling can be achieved by having a co-leader who is an older adult with arthritis in order to increase credibility with the class. If this is not possible, using a video can demonstrate desired behaviors.

Helping older adults with arthritis to reinterpret symptoms increases their self-efficacy for symptom management. When they hear about the "stress-pain-depression" cycle, they find it easier to understand how physical and emotional symptoms interact. When pain is experienced, a response is to tighten muscles in the affected area, which causes further pain. As pain increases, stress and tension increase, causing the older adult with arthritis to wonder if the pain will ever get better. A vicious cycle is created if this leads to a decrease in activities, further causing weak muscles and pain; depression can result (Lorig, 1997). As each symptom is discussed, multiple possible causes can be suggested and self-management techniques taught. Although verbal persuasion is the least effective way to increase self-efficacy, if used judiciously, it can encourage them to do a little more than they were doing last week.

Supported by research demonstrating successful outcomes, and patient satisfaction, arthritis self-management classes should be added to the nurse's repertoire of successful teaching tools and self-help techniques for older adults with arthritis.

MEDICAL IMPLICATIONS

In a summary of a National Institutes of Health (NIH) Conference on "Osteoarthritis: New Insights," Hochberg, McAlindon, and Felson (2000) state, "Major advances in management to reduce pain and disability are yielding a panoply of available treatments from nutriceuticals to chondrocyte transplantation, new oral antiinflamatory medications, and health education."(p. 726). Patient education is a cornerstone of the treatment of arthritis. However, less than 2% of the U.S. population with arthritis has participated in these interventions, even though results show that participation in these programs by people with osteoarthritis improve health status and are cost effective. Hochberg et al. conclude that one reason for the low participation rate is that these interventions have been implemented largely outside the health care system, and that until these interventions are incorporated into medical care, their benefits may go largely unrealized.

SUMMARY

Given the lack of reimbursement for health education teaching, the conclusions of the NIH Conference may represent an awful truth. The key, then, is for nurses to market self-management techniques for older adults with arthritis to the other health professionals within the system. Enlisting the support of our physician colleagues is a technique nurses sometimes overlook. The physicians barely have time for diagnosis and treatment, and even though they may be aware of the importance of patient education, there is no time to do it. Nurses need to make them aware of the benefits of arthritis self-management and to create a partnership that will benefit the patient. In *Patient Education: A Practical Approach* (Lorig, 1996), the suggestion is to make up special prescription pads (small printers can do this inexpensively). Then, in much the same way as the doctor prescribes medication, s/he could prescribe patient education. This would involve the physician in a way that would make both the patient and the physician recognize the importance of viewing arthritis self-management as a legitimate part of the treatment plan.

From a health policy perspective, the *National Arthritis Action Plan* (Centers for Disease Control and Prevention, 1999) calls upon health care providers to "develop strategies to engage people with arthritis who do not participate in self-management programs" (p. 23) and to conduct research to answer the question: "How do self-management approaches differ in different social, cultural, and economic groups?" (p. 23) and the direction to "build self-management education programs, such as the Arthritis Self-Help Course, into routine arthritis care." (p. 23). The proposed *Healthy People 2010* (U.S. Department of Health and Human Services, 1998) Arthritis-Related Objectives # 9 directs health care providers to "Increase the proportion of people with arthritis who have had effective, evidence-based arthritis education (including information about community and self-help resources) as an integral part of the management of their condition" (p. 39).

Some older adults with arthritis only need nurses' support and encouragement to manage their pain. They face their daily tasks despite pain. As one participant in the ASHC stated, "We don't want pity, just understanding; I've learned I have to help myself, let other people help me, move a little at a time, and just keep on keepin' on." Contributing to the quality of life of the courageous people who are struggling with adapting to living with arthritis is a worthy goal. Together, all health care providers can make a difference in the lives of older adults with arthritis.

Note: This research was supported by a Department of Health and Human Services National Institute of Nursing Research Grant, No. 1 R15 NR/ODO4016–01A1.

REFERENCES

Arthritis Foundation. (1997). *The arthritis self-help course.* Atlanta: Author.

Arthritis Foundation. (2000).*The Arthritis Foundation's tips for good living with arthritis.* Atlanta: Author.

Bandura, A. (1986*). Social foundations of thought and action: A social cognitive theory.* Englewood Cliffs, NJ: Prentice Hall.

Bill-Harvey, D., Rippey, R., Abeles, M., & Pfeiffer, C. (1989). Methods used by urban, low-income minorities to care for their arthritis. *Arthritis Care and Research, 2,* 60–64.

Centers for Disease Control and Prevention. (1999). *National arthritis plan: a public health strategy* Atlanta: Arthritis Foundation; Association of State and Territorial Health officials, The Agency.

Cooper, R. (1991). Celebrate diversity—or should we? *Ethnicity and Disease, 1,* 3–7.

Dennis, B., & Neese, J. (2000). Recruitment and retention of African American elders into community-based research: Lessons learned. *Archives of Psychiatric Nursing, 14,* 3–11.

Doak, C., Doak, L., & Root, J. (1996). *Teaching patients with low literacy skills.* Philadelphia: Lippincott.

Dukski, T., & Newman, A. (1989). The effectiveness of relaxation in relieving pain in women with rheumatoid arthritis. In S. Funk, E. Tournquist, M. Champagne, L. Copp, R. Weiss (Eds.), *Key aspects of comfort: Management of pain, fatigue, and nausea,* New York: Springer.

Ellison, C. (1983). Spiritual well-being: Conceptualization and measurement. *Journal of Psychology and Theology, 11,* 330–340.

Francis, C. (1992). Emerging majority suffers from poverty, lack of access, poor primary care. *Proceedings of the 4th National Forum on Cardiovascular Health, Pulmonary Disorders, and Blood Pressure.* Washington, DC.

Goeppinger, J., & Lorig, K. (1997). Interventions to reduce the impact of chronic disease: Community-based arthritis patient education. *Annual Review of Nursing Research, 15,* 101–122.

Goeppinger, J., Macnee, C., Anderson, M., Boutaugh, M., & Stewart, K. (1995). From research to practice: The effects of a jointly sponsored dissemination of an arthritis self-care nursing intervention. *Applied Nursing Research, 8,* 106–113.

Hochberg, M., McAlindon, T., & Felson, D. (2000). Systemic and topical treatments. In Felson, D. T., conference chair. Osteoarthritis: new insights. Part 2: Treatment approaches. *Annal of Internal Medicine, 133,* 726–737.

Kee, C. (2000). Osteoarthritis: Manageable scourge of aging. *Nursing Clinics of North America, 1,* 199–208.

Kumanyika, S., & Golden, P. (1991). Cross-sectional differences in health status in US racial/ethnic minority groups: Potential influences of temporal changes, disease, and life-style transitions. *Ethnicity and Disease, 1,* 50–59.

Lorig, K. (1996). *Patient education: A practical approach.* Thousand Oaks, CA: Sage.

Lorig K. (1997). *Arthritis self-help course: Leader's manual and reference material.* Atlanta, GA: The Arthritis Foundation.

Lorig, K., Chastain, R., Ung, E., Shoor, S., & Holman, H. (1989). Development and evaluation of a scale to measure the perceived self-efficacy of people with arthritis. *Arthritis and Rheumatism, 32,* 37–44.

Lorig, K., & Fries, J. (1995). *The arthritis helpbook: A tested self-management program for coping with your arthritis.* Reading, MA: Addison-Wesley.

Lorig, K., & Gonzalez, V. (1992) The integration of theory with practice: A 12–year case study. *Health Education Quarterly, 19,* 355–386.

Lorig, K., Mazonson, P., & Holman, E. (1993). Evidence suggesting that health education for self-management in patients with chronic arthritis has sustained health benefits while reducing health care costs. *Arthritis Care and Research, 2,* S8.

Lorig K Seleznick M Lubeck D. Ung E Chastain R Holman H. (1989).The beneficial outcomes of the arthritis self-management course are not adequately explained by behavior change. *Arthritis and Rheumatism,* 32:1: 91–95.

Lorig K., Mazonson, P., & Holman, H. (1989) Four year clinical and service utilization benefits of arthritis patient education. *Arthritis and Rheumatism, 36,* 439–46.

Newman, A. (1993). Effects of a self-help program on women with arthritis. In S. Funk, E. Tournquist, M. Champagne & R. Weiss (Eds.). *Key aspects of chronic pain: Hospital and home,* New York: Springer.

Newman, A. (2001). Self-help care in older African Americans with arthritis. *Geriatric Nursing, 22,* 1–4.

Nodhturft, V., Schneider, J., Herbert, P., Bradham, D., Bryant, M., Phillips, M., Russo, K., Goettelman, D., Aldahondo, A., Clark, V., & Wagener, S. (2000). Chronic disease management: Improving health outcomes. *Nursing Clinics of North America, 2,*507–518.

Stephenson, K., Yee, B., & Lisse, J. (1997). Adaptive coping skills for older African Americans with arthritis. *Topics Geriatr Rehabil, 12,* 75–87.

United States Department of Health and Human Services. (1996*). Toward equality of well-being: Strategies for improving minority health.* Washington, DC: U.S. Government Printing Office.

United States Department of Health and Human Services. (1998). *Healthy people 2010 objectives: Draft for public comment.* Washington, DC: Office of Disease Prevention and Health Promotion.

Weinert, C. (1987). A social support measure: PRQ85. *Nursing Research, 36,* 273–277.

11
Quality of Life Issues

Phyllis J. Atkinson

The World Health Organization defined quality of life as the "individual's perception of his/her position in life in the context of the culture and value systems in which one lives, and in relation to the goals, expectations, and concerns" (World Health Organization Quality of Life Group, 1993). There is no universally accepted definition for quality of life. It is a subjective experience that must be described and defined by each individual.

There are many domains that quality of life encompasses, such as physical and mental well-being and social relationships. Functional ability, spirituality, environment (adequate housing, geographically accessible to needs), and culture are other domains quality of life encompasses. While the domains can be isolated and discussed as separate entities, there is also a dynamic interaction among them (King & Hinds, 1998). Physical concerns or decreased function impact psychological well-being. Physical symptoms also can impact social and spiritual concerns.

Arthritis has a significant impact on quality of life, not only for those who experience its disabling pain but also for the caregivers. Caregivers must face a change or disruption in their lifestyle to accommodate assisting the loved one with chronic debilitating arthritis.

THE DOMAINS THAT IMPACT QUALITY OF LIFE

There are many domains that impact quality of life. Grant, Ferrell, and Sakurai (1994) identified quality of life as consisting of four dimensions/domains, which include physical well-being, psychological well-being, social well-being, and spiritual well-being. Each domain consists of specific items. Physical well-being consists of functional ability, strength/fatigue, sleep and rest, overall physical health and fertility. Psychological well-being includes maintaining self-control, avoiding anxiety, depression, interspersing enjoyment/ leisure activities, and reducing any distress of the diagnosis of arthritis. Social well-being includes family distress, roles and relationship, affection/sexual function, isolation, and finances. Spiritual well-being includes meaning of illness, religiosity, hope, uncertainty, and inner strength. Although Grant and colleagues' research focused on the impact of cancer on quality of life their model can be applied to all chronic diseases, including arthritis.

In the 1996–1998 study completed by the Centers for Disease Control and Prevention (2000), respondents with arthritis reported having fair or poor health approximately three times more often than those without arthritis. Those with arthritis averaged 4.2 more days when physical health was not good, mild symptoms that limited some physical activity 1.6 more days when mental health was not good, 4.6 more unhealthy days (actual physical illness present) and 2.3 more days of recent activity limitation because of poor physical or mental health.

The physical symptoms of arthritis such as pain, fatigue and decreased joint motion typically result in overall decreased physical activity. This inactivity has the potential to lead to further physical conditions such as obesity, hypertension, diabetes, coronary artery disease, and depression. Pain, fatigue, and decreased joint pain can limit the individuals' capacity to perform activities of daily living and instrumental activities, especially cooking, cleaning and transportation. Weight loss can be a concern secondary to loss of appetite from pain or being too fatigued and in too much pain to prepare a meal. In addition, people with arthritis may be dependent on others for transferring secondary to their limited mobility. Their increased dependence increases the burden on others as well as their own feelings of helplessness and worthlessness. Such feelings have the potential to lead to depression and anxiety.

Older adults who do not have good pain control and are physically limited due to their disease often isolate themselves. This isolation can lead to depression, anger, and anxiety. Arthritis-afflicted individuals may have difficulty coping with their disability and pain, which can also lead to increased feelings of helplessness and lack of control.

Arthritis can cause an older adult to retire early from the work force. This can have financial as well as psychological implications. In addition, the disease can place a financial burden on individuals and their loved ones secondary to the costs of health care and medications needed.

Carr (1999) found that patients with osteoarthritis perceived themselves to be handicapped in functional and social activities, relationships, socioeconomic status, emotional well-being, and body image. Similar studies revealed that social support plays an important role in moderating the effects of pain, functional limitation, and depression on the quality of life of those individuals with osteoarthritis (Blixen & Kippes, 1999). Individuals who reported the most pain were women and those who had rheumatoid arthritis, regardless of their gender (Affleck, et al., 1999). The authors found that women used more outward focused strategies and men were more likely to report an increase in negative mood associated with inward focused strategies the day after a more painful day.

ASSESSMENT

The concept of quality of life is increasingly important as a valid indicator of whether a given treatment is beneficial. There are several assessment tools that were designed primarily to determine if a particular drug makes an impact on an individual's quality of life. Some of these tools include the Health Assessment Questionnaire (HAQ), Arthritis Impact Measurement Scale (AIMS), Short Form Health Survey (SF-36), Multidimensional Health Assessment Questionnaire (MDHAQ), and the Sickness Impact Measurement Scale. Studies report whether those who receive the medication improve their quality of life.

The Health Assessment Questionnaire (HAQ) and pain assessment scores are used to quantitatively determine an individual's quality of life (Wolfe, 2001). The HAQ is a 20–item questionnaire that asks about functioning within eight categories. These categories include dressing and grooming, hygiene, arising, reach, eating, grip, walking, and activities. Each question is scored from 0–3 with 0 indicating no difficulty, 1 indicating some difficulty, 2 indicating with much difficulty or necessitating the use of an assistive device, and 3 indicating inability to perform the task. This tool can indicate a change in either direction if the scores are compared to a series of use or intervals such as annual testing.

The Arthritis Impact Measurement Scale (AIMS) was designed as an indicator of the outcome of care for arthritic patients (Meenan, Gertman, & Mason, 1980). The scale has 45 items that cover physical, social, and emotional well-being. There are an additional 19 items that cover general health and health perceptions. There is also an 18–item abbreviated version of the AIMS (Wallston, Brown, Stein, & Dobbins, 1989). The abbreviated version includes two of the best-performing items identified by the authors of the tool from each of the nine subscales in the 45–item version. The average length of time to complete the AIMS is fifteen to twenty minutes. The AIMS Short Version takes an average of six to eight minutes to complete.

Another instrument used in medical outcome studies is the Short Form Health Survey-36 (SF-36), which is considered to be a quality of life measure. It was designed to measure overall functional status and well-being for adult patients. The SF-36 measures quality of life issues in a series of domains. These domains, including physical function, bodily pain, general health, vitality, social functioning, emotional and mental health (Brazier, et al., 1992; Wolfe, 2001).

Pincus, Swearingen, and Wolfe (1999) developed the Multidimensional Health Assessment Questionnaire (MDHAQ). This assessment tool was developed through the addition of new items to the Health Assessment Questionnaire (HAQ). The new items, including advanced activities of daily living and psychological distress in routine care, were designed to capture the functional limitations of the HAQ and the Modified HAQ (MHAQ). Pincus et al. thought patients were able to report normal scores on the HAQ and MHAQ even though they may be having meaningful functional limitations. Errands, stair climbing, walking two miles, participating in sports and games, and running/jogging two miles were some of the advanced activities of daily living included on the form. The advanced MDHAQ overcame the limitations of the HAQ and MHAQ. It was found to be a useful tool to screen for problems with sleep, stress, anxiety, and depression. The questionnaire is designed in a 2–page, "patient-friendly," format. The data supported the value of using this questionnaire by each patient at each physician visit.

Carr (1999) looked at the importance of measuring the wider personal and social consequences of osteoarthritis (OA). The data suggested that the psychosocial impact of OA might have been underestimated in the past.

Through a telephone survey, the Centers for Disease Control and Prevention highlighted the burden of arthritis in the American society (2000). Their data were gathered between 1996 and 1998 from 32,322 respondents (9,899 of whom had arthritis) who resided in 11 different states. Individuals with arthritis reported significantly poorer health-related quality of life than those without arthritis. Those with arthritis were more likely to report their overall health, including physical and mental, as fair or poor and they had greater limitation in their activity level.

Social support was found to play an important role in moderating the effects of pain, functional limitation, and depression in older adults with osteoarthritis (Blixen & Kippes, 1999).

Measurement of quality of life was a focus at a conference presented by Clancy and others (Spertus, 2000). Clancy, a senior scientist at the Agency for Health Care Research and Quality, challenges health care professionals to move beyond the current "test tube" model of studying health status measures. He encourages the movement to a paradigm where health professionals routinely use tools to monitor patients' quality of life and the effect of current therapy and treatment. Clancy believes this change will enhance the quality of patient/provider communication at the time of treatment decision making.

Health care professionals should be aware of the characteristics of quality of life scales and how they differ from disease-specific instruments, such as the Arthritis Impact Measurement Scale, or general health scales, such as the Sickness Impact Profile (Strawbridge, 1998). Strawbridge believes a good quality of life scale assesses dimensions of everyday life that are missed by health-specific scales. It is imperative that health care providers determine what "quality of life" means to their individual patients.

NURSING INTERVENTIONS

Nurses play an important role in the arena of the older adult with arthritis. Nurses must not assume they know how a patient or caregiver dealing with arthritis feels or rates quality of life. In one study, King, Ferrell, Grant, and Sakurai (1995) looked at nurses' perceptions of the impact of bone marrow transplantation on the quality of life of survivors. The nurses' responses to a quality of life questionnaire were compared with the responses of the bone marrow transplant survivors. Results revealed nurses perceived patients to have a poorer quality of life than that actually reported by patients.

Using the domains that impact quality of life may be useful in guiding the formulation of nursing diagnoses. Table 11.1 has a list of appropriate nursing diagnoses.

There are practices health care professionals can implement as well as teach their patients to implement that could improve patients quality of life. The National Arthritis Action Plan is a public health strategy that was developed to serve as a guide for the fulfillment of the quality of life aspect of the Foundation's mission statement (Brady et al., 1999). It was based on documented needs and

TABLE 11.1 Nursing Diagnoses Relevant to Quality of Life Issues

Activity alteration	Activity intolerance
Activity intolerance risk	Activities of daily living Alteration
Acute pain	Adjustment impairment
Anxiety	Bathing/hygiene deficit
Body nutrition deficit	Chronic pain
Compromised family coping	Disabled family coping
Disuse syndrome	Dressing/grooming deficit
Family coping impairment	Fatigue
Fear	Hopelessness
Individual coping impairment	Meaningfulness alteration
Physical mobility impairment	Polypharmacy
Powerlessness	Role performance alteration
Self care deficit	Sexuality patterns alteration
Social isolation	Socialization alteration

challenges that affect quality of life, with a focus on physical, psychosocial and economic issues. The plan should guide the use of the nation's resources to decrease the burden of arthritis for all Americans and increase the quality of life of those affected by arthritis.

The National Arthritis Action Plan outlined primary, secondary, and tertiary prevention strategies. Primary prevention strategies include identifying through research and educating the public and health care professionals about the factors that increase the risk of arthritis. The secondary prevention strategies include early diagnosis and medical treatment. These strategies are underused because many individuals do not seek medical attention for their arthritis when there is minimal limitation of their activities. The tertiary prevention strategies are those that can reduce pain and disability, increase a person's sense of control, and improve quality of life.

An example of a tertiary prevention strategy is self-management. Self-management techniques include weight control, promotion of physical activity, education, about the disease, nutrition, patient-provider communication, medications, relaxation and pain-management techniques, self-care skills, and physical and occupational therapy.

The National Institute of Arthritis and Musculoskeletal and Skin Disease's publication, *Osteoarthritis* (NIH, 1998) discusses adopting a "good-health attitude." A good-health attitude includes (1) encouraging your patients to focus on their abilities and strengths instead of their disabilities and weaknesses; (2) teaching your patients methods of breaking down their activities into small tasks that they can manage in an effort to balance rest with activity while incorporating fitness and nutrition into their daily routines; (3) teaching your patients methods to reduce and manage stress; and, (4) helping your patients develop a support system of family, friends, and health professionals. Individuals with arthritis who participate in self-care are usually more successful in managing their pain and the disability of the disease. Providing educational information about the disease and encouraging patients to be important members of the health care team will enable them to decrease their level of pain and feel an enhanced sense of control over their lives.

As previously stated, arthritis not only affects the patients' quality of life but also those caring for them. Health care providers should ensure that caregivers receive the support and respite needed.

CONCLUSION

Identifying how and what each individual patient defines as quality of life is essential. Is it being free from pain, fixing oneself dinner, playing with grandchildren, working, bathing, and dressing oneself, or is it something entirely different? Healthcare professionals cannot know unless they ask. We need to ask important questions such as what is the most important thing in your life? What makes you happy? What makes you sad? What are your goals for the future? These are simple, yet very powerful questions that can enable healthcare providers to better define an individual's quality of life.

Staying abreast of all the modalities/interventions/strategies that have been shown to decrease the disability and pain associated with arthritis is key to improving the quality of life of individuals with the disabling disease. The National Arthritis Action Plan (Brady et al., 1999) is a detailed guide to improving the quality of life for individuals with arthritis. As providers to individuals with this disease we have a responsibility to embrace the plan and begin improving the quality of life for those we serve.

REFERENCES

Affleck, G., Tennen, H., Keefe, F., Lefebvre, J., Kashikar-Zuck, S., Wright, K., Starr, K., & Caldwell, D. (1999). Everyday life with osteoarthritis or rheumatoid arthritis: Independent effects of disease and gender on daily pain, mood, and coping. *Pain, 83*(3), 601–609.

Blixen, C., & Kippes, C. (1999). Depression, social support, and quality of life in older adults with osteoarthritis. *Image. 31*(3), 221–226.

Bonomi, A., Shikiar, R., & Legro, M., 2000. Quality of life assessment in acute, chronic and cancer pain, A pharmacist's guide. *Journal of the American Pharmaceutical Association, 40*(3), 402–416.

Brady, T., Conn, D., Foneska, J., Meenan, R., Alongi, J., Gay, M., Harris, A., Helmick, C., Hogelin, G., Holt, J., & Smith, S. (1999). National Arthritis Action Plan: A public Health Strategy. Available at *www.arthritis.org/answers/about-naap.asp*

Brazier, J., Harper, R., Jones, N., O'Cathain, A., Thomas, K., Usherwood, T., Westlake, L. (1992). Validating the SF-36 Health Survey Questionnaire: New outcome measure for primary care. *British Medical Journal, 305*(6846), 160–164.

Carr, A. (1999). Beyond disability: Measuring the social and personal consequences of osteoarthritis. *Osteoarthritis Cartilage, 7*(2), 230–238.

Centers for Disease Control and Prevention. (2000). Health-related quality of life among adults with arthritis-behavioral risk factor surveillance system, 11 states, 1996–1998. *Morbidity and Mortality Weekly Report, 49,* 366.

Grant, M., Ferrell, B., & Sakurai, C. (1994). Defining the spiritual dimension of quality of life assessment in bone marrow transplant survivors. *Oncology Nursing Forum, 21*(2), 376.

King, C., Ferrell, B. R., Grant, M., & Sakurai, C. (1995). Nurses' perceptions of the meaning of quality of life for bone marrow transplant survivors. *Cancer Nursing, 18,* 118–129.

King, C., & Hinds, P. (1998). *Quality of life, from nursing and patient perspectives.* Boston: Jones & Bartlett.

Meenan, R., Gertman, P., Mason, J., (1980). Measuring health status in arthritis: The Arthritis Impact Measurement Scales. *Arthritis and Rheumatism, 23*(2), 146–152.

National Institutes of Health: National Institute of Arthritis and Musculoskeletal and Skin Disease. (1998). *Osteoarthritis.* NIH Publication No. 99–4617. Washington, DC: Author.

Pincus, T., Swearingen, C., & Wolfe, F. (1999). Toward a multidimensional Health Assessment Questionnaire (MDHAQ): Assessment of advanced activities of daily living and psychological status in the patient-friendly health assessment questionnaire format. *Arthritis Rheumatology, 42*(10), 2220–2230.

Spertus, J., 2000. Measuring quality of life and functional status. From an April 10, 2000 session at the AHA/ACC 2nd Scientific Forum on Quality of Care and Outcomes Research in Cardiovascular Disease and Stroke, presented by C. Clancy, J. Cooper, S. Dunbar, J. Spertus, F. Wolinsky, & K. Wyrwich, W. Strawbridge. Feb. 8, 1998. Quality of life: What is it and can it be measured? *Growth Hormone IGF Research* (Supplement A), 59–62.

Strawbridge, W. (1998). Quality of life: What is it and can it be measured. *Growth Hormone IGF Research,* (8) suppl. A, pp. 59-62.

Wallston, K., Brown, G., Stein, M., Dobbins, C. (1989). Comparing the short and long versions of the Arthritis Impact Measurement Scales. *Journal of Rheumatology, 16*(8), 1105-1109.

Wolfe, F. (2001). Correlation between progression of joint damage and long-term outcomes including functional quality of life and disability: The impact of anti-TNF-a therapy. Available at *www.medscape.com/CMECircle/rheumatology/2001/CME01/pnt-CME01.html*

World Health Organization Quality of Life Group. (1993). Study protocol for the World Health Organization project to develop a quality of life assessment instrument (the WHOQOL). *Quality of Life Research, 2,* 153–159.

12
Alternative and Complementary Therapies

Mary R. Painter-Romanello

Currently, there is an increasing dissatisfaction with the effectiveness of conventional medicine, particularly in treating chronic diseases (Spencer & Jacobs, 1999). Because arthritis is a common chronic complaint among older adults, alternative therapies are frequently being investigated. A survey of patients in a rheumatology clinic revealed a 61% utilization of alternative therapies with an average of 2.5 therapies/patient (Cauffield, 2000). Those diagnosed with rheumatoid arthritis were more likely to use alternative therapies (38%) compared with those who had osteoarthritis (23%). In a study looking at the use of alternative therapies by older adults with osteoarthritis (Ramsey, Spencer, Topolski, Belza, & Patrick, 2001) 47% of participants reported using at least one type of alternative care during a 20–week intervention period. Clearly, this is an area of concern for nurses who manage care for this older age group.

DEFINITION

Complementary and alternative medicine (CAM) is the term used to describe non-traditional means of treatment. The intent of these treatments is to provide care with a mind/body/spirit approach that addresses health concerns within the context of total well-being (Snyder & Lindquist, 1998). Within the past decade, these methods have become increasingly popular in the United States in spite of the fact they are costly, rarely covered by insurance, and there is little in the way of substantial research data to support their use (Kramer, 1999).

DISCUSSION

Central to all alternative therapies is the patient's/practitioner's belief system. Each therapy is individualized and designed to empower individuals to be accountable for their own health. Practitioners of alternative therapies will inform patients that they must be active participants in their care and that they are expected to eventually assume responsibility for incorporation of the therapies into their lives (Snyder & Lindquist, 1998). In addition, it is imperative the use of these modalities be shared with an individual's primary care provider. Only half of CAM users tell their physicians about their use of alternative therapies (Cauffield, 2000). These therapies can also involve considerable time and financial commitments. CAM users spent an out of pocket $21.2—32.7 billion versus $29.3 billion for medical treatment (Cauffield, 2000).

Prior to initiating any alternative therapy, a complete physical should be done to identify serious conditions. All health histories should include questions about alternative therapies, including the use of herbals and supplements. However, these issues must be addressed in an objective, nonjudgmental manner so as to encourage patient disclosure (Cauffield, 2000).

ALTERNATIVE THERAPIES

The following CAM therapies are the most commonly used for arthritis:

- Chiropractic
- Acupuncture

- Relaxation/mind—body therapies
- Tai Chi/Yoga
- Dietary supplements/herbals/homeopathic

Chiropractic Treatments

Chiropractic treatments are focused on specific joints to relax surrounding tissue, improve circulation and improve joint flexibility. In addition, the effects of diet, exercise, rest, stress, and environment are evaluated. One study of older adults with osteoarthritis found that chiropractic services were used by 20.7% of the subjects (Ramsey, et al., 2001). The results of a second study endorse the use of chiropractic services as an effective and conservative approach to osteoarthritis treatment (Gottlieb, 1997).

Acupuncture

Acupuncture is part of traditional Chinese medicine (TCM) in which ultrafine needles are inserted into various "points" on the body in order to improve the flow of the life force, or *qi*. The National Institutes of Health (NIH), in a 1997 consensus statement, noted acupuncture to be a reasonable adjunctive pain management option for osteoarthritis (Del Rosario, 2001). However, the American College of Rheumatology (2001) reported that acupuncture works no better than placebo. To help resolve conflicts such as this, the Center for Alternative Medicine Evaluation and Research in Arthritis (CAMRA, 2001) has been developed at the University of Maryland, Baltimore. The center explores the potential efficacy, safety, and cost effectiveness of alternative therapies for arthritis and related diseases (Berman, Hartnoll & Bausell, 2000). Currently, they have a study to determine the safety and efficacy of acupuncture in knee osteoarthritis. Others are planned to follow (CAMRA, 2001).

Relaxation/Mind-Body Therapies

The most well-known relaxation/mind-body therapies are meditation, imagery, and biofeedback. The goal is to place a person in a deep restful state that reduces the body's stress response. Continued practice allows the person to achieve relaxed breathing, slowed brain waves, and decreased muscle tension and heart rate. Each of these has been shown to be successful in decreasing chronic pain, which can benefit an older adult with arthritis (Snyder & Lindquist, 1998). However, these therapies require patience and possibly a different individualized approach, which might take longer for an older person with other established coping mechanisms.

Tai Chi and Yoga

Tai chi and yoga are two movement therapies shown to be beneficial to older adults who have arthritis (Chen & Snyder, 1999; Garfinkel & Schumacher, 2000). Both focus on relaxation of the entire body through systematic movement in coordination with deep breathing (Snyder & Lindquist, 1998). The slow, deliberate movements are not difficult for older adults and after a period of time, measurable improvements can be seen in balance, strength, and flexibility, thus preserving functional status, an important consideration for an older adult with arthritis (Snyder & Lindquist, 1998).

Dietary Supplements, Herbals, and Homeopathic

An area of fast growing CAM practices is the use of nutritional supplements, herbal products, and homeopathic remedies. There are currently more than 800 companies producing medicinal plant products with annual revenues in excess of $4.5 billion (Cauffield 2000; Murch, KrishnaRaj, & Saxena, 2000). However, numerous problems have arisen that have compromised the quality, safety, and efficacy of these products, including variability in crop and product quality; variability in the concentration of phytomedicine's active components; adulteration of medicinal preparations with misidentified plant species; contamination of plant materials with insects, bacteria and fungi; lack of understanding of the efficacy with human consumption; and consumer fraud. In addition, the identity of the active constituent in a plant is not easily identified, and concentrations of active and marker constituents have a high degree of variability from plant to plant (Murch, KrishnaRaj, & Saxena, 2000).

A survey of 176 patients from a geriatric rheumatology clinic revealed that 66% used some form of alternative medicines (Anderson, Shane-McWhorter, Crouch, & Andersen, 2000). Most thought that the agents were safe and took them because they believe they have added benefits. The use of alternative medicines increased with number of diagnoses and greater perceived safety of the products. However, herbal medicines are not without risk. Adverse effects include allergic reactions, liver function abnormalities, hypertension, and psychosis. Certain people, including elderly patients, are at high risk of toxicity and/or drug interactions, necessitating thorough drug histories about herbals, supplements and homeopathic (Andersen, et al., 2000; Fetrow & Avila, 1999).

A dietary supplement, as defined in the Dietary Supplement Health and Education Act (DSHEA) of 1994, is a product taken by mouth that contains a "dietary ingredient" intended to supplement the diet. It must be one or any combination of the following:

- a vitamin
- a mineral
- an herb or other botanical
- an amino acid
- an enzyme or tissue from organs or glands
- a concentrate, metabolite, constituent, or extract

Dietary supplements are not regulated, or approved by the Federal Drug Administration (FDA) and there are no FDA regulations that establish a minimum standard of practice for manufacturing them. The manufacturer is responsible for determining that its product is safe and that any representations or claims made are substantiated by adequate evidence (U.S. Food and Drug Administration, 2001).

Tables 12.1 and 12.2 provide some recommended supplements for osteoarthritis and rheumatoid arthritis. Each has specific considerations and contraindications as well as condition-specific dosages and should be thoroughly investigated prior to use (Fetrow & Avila, 1999; Grant & Lutz, 2000; Grant & Schneider, 2000; LaValle, Krinsky, Hawkins, Pelton & Willis, 2000).

TABLE 12.1 Supplements for Osteoarthritis

Herb	Vitamin/Mineral/ Trace Element/ Nutraceutical	Homeopathic Remedy	Additional Supplements
Boswellia	Chondroitin Sulfate, Glucosamine Sulfate, or Glucosamine Hydrochloride	Arnica Montana	Boron
Ginger	Methyl Sulfonyl Methane (MSM)	Bryonia alba	
Grape Seed	SAMe (S-adenosylmethionine)	Calcarea phosphorica	
Cat's Claw	Collagen	Dulcamara	
Tumeric		Rhus toxicodendron	

TABLE 12.2 Supplements for Rheumatoid Arthritis

Herb	Vitamin/Mineral/ Trace Element/ Nutraceutical	Homeopathic Remedy	Additional Supplements
Cat's Claw	Shark Cartilage	Apis mellifica	Boron
Boswellia	Methyl Sulfonyl Methane (MSM)	Arnica Montana	Fish Oils, or Flaxseed Oil
Devil's Claw	Collagen	Causticum	
Evening Primose	Chondroitin Sulfate, Glucosamine Sulfate, or Glucosamine Hydrochloride	Colchicum autumnale	
Turmeric	Vitamin B_5	Ledum palustre	
Bromelain	Vitamin E Copper Salicylate	Rhus toxicodendron	

SUMMARY

CAM therapies for the older adult with arthritis include a variety of modalities. Although many have anecdotal success, there are a limited number of studies to support them. In spite of this, the growth in CAM has been consumer driven, largely due to dissatisfaction with current medical treatment. Alternative therapies allow for unique, individualized treatments that affect the whole person, not just a symptom.

Those therapies with the most significant supporting evidence are nutritional supplements, particularly glucosamine, herbs, and acupuncture. Those with moderate supporting evidence include yoga, relaxation, and chiropractic, and the least supported therapies are tai chi, guided imagery, and meditation (Spencer & Jacobs, 1999).

REFERENCES

American College of Rheumatology. (2001). Complementary and alternative medicine. *http://mayoclinic.com/home?id=HQO1121*

Andersen, D. L., Shane-McWhorter, L., Crouch, B. I., Andersen, S. J. (2000). Prevalence and patterns of alternative medication use in a university hospital outpatient clinic serving rheumatology and geriatric patients. *Pharmacotherapy, 20*(8), 958–966.

Berman, B. M., Hartnoll, S., Bausell, B. (2000). CAM evaluation comes into the mainstream: NIH specialized Centers of Research and the University of Maryland Center for Alternative Medicine Research in Arthritis. *Complementary Therapies in Medicine, 8*(2):119–22.

Cauffield, J. S. (2000) The psychosocial aspects of complementary and alternative medicine. *Pharmacotherapy, 20*(11), 1289–1294.

CAMRA (Center for Alternative Medicine Research of Arthritis). (2000). *http://www.clinical* trials.gov

Chen, K. M., Snyder, M. (1999). A research-based use of Ti Chi/movement therapy as a nursing intervention. *Journal of Holistic Nursing, 17*(3), 267–79.

DelRosario, J. (2001). Acupuncture as alternative therapy. *Advance for Providers of Post-Acute Care, 4*(3), 30–31 & 81.

Fetrow, C. W., & Avila, J. R.(1999). *Professional's handbook of complementary & alternative medicines.* Springhouse, PA: Springhouse.

Garfinkel M., & Schumacher, H. R., Jr. (2000). Yoga. *Rheumatology Disease Clinics of North America, 26*(1), 125–32,x.

Gottlieb, M. S. (1997). Conservative management of spinal osteoarthritis with glucosamine sulfate and chiropractic treatment. *Journal of Manipulative Physiological Therapeutics 1997, 20*(6), 400–414.

Grant, K., & Lutz, R. B. (2000). Alternative therapies: Ginger. *American Journal of Health-System Pharmacy, 57*(10), 945–947

Grant, K. & Schneider, C. D. (2000). Alternative therapies: Turmeric. *American Journal of Health-System Pharmacy, 57*(12), 1121–1122.

Kramer, N. (1999) Why I would not recommend complementary or alternative therapies: a physician's perspective. *Rheumatology Disease Clinics of North America, 25*(4), 833–43.

LaValle, J. B., Krinsky, D. L., Hawkins, E. B., Pelton, R., & Willis, N. A. (2000). *Natural therapeutics pocket guide.* Hudson OH: Lexi-comp.

Murch, S. J., KrishnaRaj, S., Saxena, P. K. (2000). Phytopharmaceuticals: Mass-production, standardization, and conservation. *Scientific Review of Alternative Medicine, 4*(2), 32–37.

Ramsey, S. D., Spencer, A. C., Topolski, T. D., Belza, B., & Patrick, D. L. (2001). Use of alternative therapies by older adults with osteoarthritis. *Arthritis and Rhematology, 45*(3), 222–227.

RCT: Acupuncture safety/efficacy in knee osteoarthritis. *http://www. clinicaltrials.gov,* 2001.

Snyder, M., & Lindquist, R.(1998). *Complementary/alternative therapies in nursing* (3rd ed.). New York: Springer.

Spencer, J. W., & Jacobs, J. J. (1999). Complementary/alternative medicine: An evidence-based approach. St. Louis: Mosby.

U.S. Food and Drug Administration, Center for Food Safety and Applied Nutrition. (2001, January 3). *Overview of dietary supplements.* Washington DC: The Agency.

13
Participating in Sports with Arthritis

Catherine A. Hill

The recent trends in exercise, leisure activities, and competitive sports for older adults invalidate the myth of the "golden years" as a time of inactivity and confinement (Hill, 2001). Eighty-five percent of seniors are reporting their health as good, very good, or excellent (Schick & Schick, 1994). Physical activities of various types are engaged in by more than 60% of adults aged 65 and older, according to the 2000 data in *Healthy People 2010* (U.S. Department of Health and Human Services, 1999). Exercise and sports choices are significant factors in how well we age (Hill). The evaluation and counseling of senior sports participants requires an understanding of senescence, arthritis pathophysiology and common injuries. A knowledge of participants' past medical history and the choice of exercise, leisure, or sport activities (Schick & Schick) is central to predicting, preventing, and treating injuries in the aging athlete. Nursing and medicine professionals are equally suited to undertake these tasks.

The national senior sports classic known as the Senior Olympics (which began in 1987) identified that 71% of senior athletes competing in 1997 began fitness activity after age 50. Women were more likely than men to embark on competitive sports after age 50 (Cornoni-Huntley, Huntley, & Feldman, 1990). In 1997, Arizona hosted

10,288 older athletes at the National Senior Sports Classic VI, who competed in 18 different sports for gold, silver, or bronze medals. A commitment to fitness can begin at any age and the choice of sport, leisure, or exercise activity is important in predicting and treating injuries in the aging athlete (Scott, 1996).

Although chronic conditions, such as arthritis (47.7% of seniors) and heart disease (59.8% of seniors), frequently occur in this age group, they are not contraindications to regular activity, especially the continuation of modified forms of prior exercise (Scott, 1996). Long-term exercise does not appear to cause excessive joint disease, and it reduces systolic and diastolic blood pressure, and improves blood lipid profiles. Fall risk and injury occur less often in older adults who participate in resistance training.

SPORTS AND POPULAR PHYSICAL ACTIVITIES DEFINED

Sports participation in the elderly is not a single entity but a collection of leisure time activities, sports participation, and conditioning exercise. Aerobic, strength, endurance and flexibility activity in older adults, in addition to the traditional measures of Activities of Daily Living (ADL) and Instrumental Activities of Daily Living (IADL) (USDHHS, 1999) are legitimate types of physical activity. Technically, leisure time physical activities are a subset of general exercise patterns and typically include gardening, dancing, golf, hunting, fishing, tennis, bowling, biking, swimming, and woodworking (USDHHS, 1999). The intensity of participation tends to be less than in exercise and competitive sports but helps maintain fitness nonetheless. In older athletes, focus is more on individual efforts than on team sports, such as long-distance running. Adults older than 50 report significantly more walking for physical activity than younger people (Dishman, 1984).

Competitive sports are an interesting new trend with seniors. These athletes are running fast and jumping high. Archery, badminton, basketball, bowling, cycling, golf, horseshoes, race-walking, racquetball, softball, swimming, table tennis, track and field, and volleyball in addition to the stereotypical shuffleboard, promote healthy lifestyles for seniors through sports and fitness (Morris, 1997). The competitive aspect of comparing one's performance against an existing norm or a competitor's is cited as very important by two thirds of the senior athletes (Fontane & Hurd, 1992).

Today we define and monitor senior exercise regimens as aerobic or strength, endurance, and flexibility training in addition to the traditional measures of activities of daily living (ADL) and instrumental. Aerobic exercise includes light, moderate, or vigorous physical activity for at least 30 minutes per day five or more times per week. In 1999, 30% of seniors met this definition(USDHHS, 1996). Strength, endurance, and flexibility training include a combination of components that improve ADL performance, functional independence, and social integration. Resistance training is particularly important for musculoskeletal health, fitness, and athletic performance (Feigenbaum & Gentry, 2001). Although traditional weight training can increase muscle strength and endurance, practically speaking other activities can accomplish the same goals for older people. The most important variable associated with risk of adverse event while exercising is the person's normal activity pattern (Vander, 1982).

INFLUENCE OF SENESCENCE VARIABILITY

The variability of senescence and the range of physical activity levels seen in elder athletes make the physiology of aging important in their assessment and treatment. Musculoskeletal and cardiovascular systems have intrinsic changes related to aging, some of which are slowed by fitness activities, whereas others may increase and affect speed of recovery from injury. The interplay of these systems often is measured by maximum oxygen consumption (VO2 max) to quantify cardiopulmonary endurance as a marker of fitness. As people age past their thirties, their maximum work capacity declines at a rate of about 1% per year (Williams, 1999). A person's highest level of conditioning influences his or her final level of decline. Therefore, athletes and untrained or sedentary seniors will have very different functional abilities. Unfortunately, the inactive senior will decline twice as fast as his counterpart (Rodeheffer, 1984).

Negative musculoskeletal changes, like cardiopulmonary changes, can be minimized by fitness training that includes sensible strength and endurance programs. However, given the physical loading forc-

TABLE 13.1 Musculoskeletal System Changes After Age 50 (Rowe, 1990)

Increased body fat
Decrease of up to 35% in lean body/muscle mass
Loss of bone mass: men 0.4% per year, women 1–7% per year
Decreased flexibility due to increased muscle collagen
Strength decrease of 10% per 10 years
Fifty percent decrease in type II (fast twitch) muscle fibers
Fifty percent decrease in ligament tensile strength
Loss of tendon glycosaminoglycan yields stiffer tendons
Decreased type XI articular cartilage
Lower articular chondroitin sulfate/chondrocyte content decreases cartilage strength
Decreased collagen water content decreases flexibility
Loss of intervertebral spinal disc water/cells/protein

es involved in most sports activities, musculoskeletal injuries are most common in the aging athlete. An understanding of senescence and knowledge of common sports injuries allows us to effectively help the aging athlete. The difference between Gordie Howe, a hockey star, playing exhibition games in his seventies, and your typical nursing home resident is the result not only of good genetics but life choices in fitness activities (Rodeheffer, 1984). Table 13.1 summarizes the physiological changes that affect the balance of fitness activity benefits versus injury risk after age 50.

ARTHRITIS AND SENIOR SPORTS

Older individuals who have remained active throughout their lives maintain much of their strength and stamina. Regardless of the age or initial fitness level of the participants, these activities should be assessed, encouraged, and monitored because of their physical and psychological benefits. The benefits and risks of regular exercise in older and elderly adults are similar to those in comparably fit younger people.

Osteoarthritis, practically universal on x-ray in at least some joints in people over age 60 years, seldom (10% to 20%) involves significant clinical disease (Pavelka, 1995). Knee disease is about twice as prevalent as hip disease in older adults (about 10% vs. 5%) (Gaffney,

1995; Pavelka, 1995). Both exercise and education have reduced pain and disability in people with osteoarthritis without causing harm. This finding compares favorably to studies of knee surgery outcomes in old age (Dieppe, Chard, Failkner, & Luhmander, 2000).

Osteoarthritis, typically defined by radiological criteria rather than clinical features, is characterized by focal areas of damage to cartilage surfaces in synovial joints and mild inflammation. Frequently osteoarthritis is an asymmetric, mono- or oligioarthropathy found in weight-bearing or overused joints. Severe osteoarthritis involves characteristic joint space narrowing and osteophyte formation, which is usually preceded by joint shape abnormality or injury. X-ray evaluation of questionable joints will allow specific staging of disease severity. According to private practice physician Warren A. Scott, pre-existing arthritis can be compounded by overuse injuries, especially in the lower extremities in the 50- to 80-year-old population (Scott, 1996). No evidence exists to prove that moderate exercise like biking, skiing, rowing, swimming, or golf increases the risk of developing osteoarthritis, according to research by Dr. J. A. Crick presented in Geriatric Grand Rounds in 1999.

The minority of elders with clinical disease of the hip or knee joint progress to surgery (Dieppe et al., 2000), and disease management is aimed at reducing the frequency and severity of activity-related and night pain, functional impairment, and progressive joint damage. These parameters will guide the modification of sports activity for older adults. Although not commonly used in the U. S., the Western Ontario and McMaster osteoarthritis index (WOMAC) is a disease-specific validated tool that is sensitive to changes in hip and knee arthritis (Bellamy, Buchanan, & Goldsmith, 1988). Recent random controlled trials reinforce the belief that exercise regimens are beneficial in reducing pain and disability (Van Baar, Assendelft, & Dekker, 1999). Changing activities from weight-bearing to non-weight-bearing, use of alternating cold and hot compresses (Meeusen, Van Der Veen, & Harley, 2001) and reducing the intensity of sports activity is recommended to manage flares of osteoarthritis pain in the aging athlete.

The use of adaptive equipment such as shoe wedges/insoles, joint braces, and joint taping to support or modify the weight distribution/loading through the joint has not been well documented in the literature. However, valgus knee bracing either by taping, neoprene sleeve or unloader-brace significantly reduces pain (by 25%) according to the two random control trials and several observational studies in current literature. (Cushnaghan, McCarthy, & Dieppe, 1994; Kirkley, Websterboggert, & Litchfield, 1999). These concepts and interventions based on the "wear and tear" pathology of osteoarthritis do not offer the same benefits to rheumatoid arthritis (RA) patients.

Luckily, the prevalence of RA is low: 0.5% to 1.5% of the general population and 10% in persons over age 65 (Schumacher, Klippel, & Koopman, 1993); however 50% of rheumatoid arthritis patients will be disabled within 10 years (Yelin, Henke, & Epstein, 1987). In contrast to osteoarthritis, rheumatoid arthritis is characterized by a chronic inflammation and its onset after age 60 is unusual (Dambro, 1998). Thus, it is the pathophysiology of rheumatoid arthritis as a symmetric polyarthropathy of smaller joints with associated systemic symptoms that dictates a different from normal approach to sports, exercise, and leisure activity, especially in the older adult. Usually treated with disease-modifying antirheumatic drugs to prevent disease progression and manage episodic flares of inflammation, articular deformities are more frequent and pronounced.

In sports activities, substantial loading forces affect each joint. If the forces are too great the tissue will fracture or tear, especially when loading stress is not absorbed by the surrounding muscles, tendons, and ligaments. Because the cartilage is so thin, most loading pressure is transmitted directly into the bone, making high impact activities high risk. The stability of joints also affects the risk in exercising older adults. Normal joints are designed to fit closely together during use, allowing the bones to bear most of the body weight. But ligament, muscles, tendons, and joint fluid also play significant roles. Since RA affects all these structures joint deformities can easily occur, making no- or low-impact activities desirable. Fatigue and decreased endurance are frequent symptoms in RA patients, both of which affect sports participation (Schumacher et al., 1993). Baseline measures of morning stiffness duration, number of affected joints, and level of pain on a scale of 1 to 10 (Dambro, 1998) will guide the patient and healthcare provider in the identification of an acute disease flare.

The traditional pyramid approach (Schumacher et al., 1993) to RA therapy is based on a combination of education, rest, and exercise, with the addition of medicines coming afterward. For seniors with good range of motion, muscle strength, and minimal joint pain, low-resistance, high-repetition activities are most appropriate. Bicycling, skiing, golfing, walking and swimming have been shown to be safe for RA patients (Schumacher et al., 1993). Patient education is vital and the American Rheumatism Association (1–800–282–7023) or the Arthritis Foundation (1–800–283–7800) are recommended as resources for the health care provider as well as the senior.

Generally, full activity in ADLs and IADLs is encouraged unless disease activity increases to cause an acute flare up of joint inflammation. The aging athlete should be advised that rest, heat, and protection of the affected joints are the rule during flares of pain, swelling, erythema and stiffness. Research shows that rest is an effective anti-inflammatory measure (Schumacher et al., 1993). Bursitis, tendinitis, and tenosynovitis can be a part of a rheumatoid arthritis flare or can be caused by trauma and chronic irritation. When the pain of an acute RA flare subsides, broad range-of-motion exercise can be resumed. Applying heat before exercise may be helpful in reducing stiffness. Mild pain (2–3 on a scale of 1–10) at the time of exercising is to be expected, especially after an area has been at rest for some time. Acute pain that lasts more than 30 minutes signals excessive exercise, disease flareup or injury.

Found more frequently in men over 60, then in other groups, gouty arthritis will produce a chronic arthritis in 50% of untreated patients (Dambro, 1998), so the initial hyperacute monoarticular inflammatory crystal arthropathy must be treated with an eye toward avoiding future problems. Control of the acute attack will require the older sports participant to rest the affected joint. Unaffected joints may be used without restriction. Use of warm and cold compresses will help the painful joint, and special attention to skin care at the site will prevent additional trauma to the inflamed joint.

Addressing the underlying cause of either overproduction or undersecretion of urate is generally successful with ongoing medication. Risk factors of obesity and hypertension make continuation of exercise and sports participation desirable. Important to the concept of accommodation is the avoidance of "all-or-nothing" thinking as it relates to the aging athlete's participation. Often a temporary change of sport or adoption of a localized workout will maintain activity levels while resting the affected joint.

Postmenopausal and involutional osteoporosis converge after age 75 (Ross, 1996) to produce increased risk for the aging athlete especially those who engage in more rigorous forms of sports. Older adults should have their bone mineral density evaluated by DEXA scan if they are 75 years old, have significant signs and symptoms, or demonstrate risk factors. Low-impact exercise, such as walking one mile twice a day is recommended (Wallach, 1998) to reduce bone loss in the treatment of osteoporosis. Continuation and modification of an aging athlete's regimen is the desired approach to a new diagnosis as well as an existing one. For the osteoporotic senior sports participant, fall precautions take on added importance and should include special attention to proper postural alignment and good body mechanics.

COMMON INJURIES

According to a 1990 report from the U. S. Consumer Product Safety Commission, which samples the National Electronic Injury Surveillance System, Americans are remaining physically active into their seventies, eighties, and nineties. In actual numbers there were 34,000 sports injuries in the 65 and older age group; the number rose to 53,000 in 1996. This 56% increase is quite a contrast to the 18% increase of sports injuries in the 25 to 64 age group. Interestingly, sports injuries increased less (29%) for people 75 and older than for people 65 to 74 years old!

Injuries from leisure activities such as fishing, golf, bowling, and shuffleboard have remained relatively constant. Golf and tennis are the most common sports played by American elders. These sports produce many of the rotator cuff tears encountered in ambulatory care (Kahn & House, 1989; Scott & Couzens, 1996). A fascinating but small number of injuries were seen for the first time in 1996 involving such "extreme" sports as snowboarding and in-line skating for older adults. Predictably, 60% of geriatric sports injuries in both 1990 and 1996 occurred in men according to a U. S. Consumer Product Safety Commission Report.

Studies of senior runners reveal an acceleration of preexisting disease with continued running. Likewise previous joint injury or abnormal joint alignment increases the risk of degenerative joint disease. Given that most elders have some x-ray evidence of arthritis of the

TABLE 13.2 Common Overuse Sports Injuries

Injury	Symptom	Likely Resulting Problem
No specific injury	Ongoing ache, improves with rest	Suspect overuse
Repetitive use of elbow	Pain increases with use, forearm/hand fatigue	Suspect tennis or golfer's elbow (tendinitis)
Chronic running or jumping activity	Anterior tibial aching, worse with use	Suspect shin splints
Chronic walking/running	Pain supralateral maleolus or lateral dorsum of foot	Suspect stress fracture
Change in activity routine or intensity	Plantar heel pain	Suspect heel spur, bruise, fascitis
Increased toeing off activity	Pain plantar surface great toe	Suspect sesmoiditis or turf toe

hip or knee and 81% of aging athletes injure themselves, moderation is critical to injury avoidance. Table 13.2 lists the common overuse injuries, their symptoms and the likely resulting problem.

While you may be familiar with fall risk in the elderly, the aging athlete will challenge the way you think of falls. From 1990 to 1996, bicycling injuries were a frequent cause for emergency room visits among all ages, 60% of which were the result of falls and 21% due to head injuries, according to the National Electronic Injury Surveillance System. Bike related injuries increased an amazing 75% in the elderly from 1990 to 1996 according to the U. S. Consumer Product Safety Commission.

Common sports fall injuries, their mechanisms, presenting symptoms, and the likely resulting problems are detailed in Table 13.3(Abdenour & Thygerson, 1993).

"Playing through the pain" is commonly engaged in by long time sports participants. This is especially worrisome in the aging athlete. Overlooking a serious injury can complicate treatment and produce chronic pain. "FOOSH" (fall on outstretched hand) occurs in nearly all sports and can lead to some of the more serious injuries (Hizon,

TABLE 13.3 Common Fall Related Sports Injuries

Injury	Symptom	Likely Resulting Problem
Fall on, twisted shoulder	Visible deformity, severe pain	Suspect dislocation, fracture
Fall on outstretched arm (FOOSH)	Can't move arm, severe pain	Suspect fracture or severe sprain/strain of clavicle/arm/wrist
Fall on shoulder, sudden throw	Felt pop, tenderness, pain	Suspect sprain, strain, contusion
Fall with hip pain	Severe pain, shortened & rotated leg	Suspect hip fracture
Fall onto or twisting of elbow	Severe pain, deformity, numbness, no rom	Suspect dislocated elbow
Fall onto elbow	Burning, tingling to hand or fingers	Suspect nerve contusion
Sudden start or stop of leg	Infracalf pain, pop at time of injury, difficulty weight bearing	Suspect Achilles tendon tear
Ankle twisting	Pain/ecchymosis lateral inframaleolus	Suspect sprain

2001). Diffuse hand pain and pain on palpation of the anatomical snuffbox along the radial aspect of the hand should trigger suspicion of scaphoid fracture and an x-ray with a "scaphoid view" which is repeated two to four weeks post fall. Failure to recognize and treat this injury can lead to nonunion and chronic lifelong pain because of degenerative joint disease. Radial head fracture is another injury often difficult to identify even with timely radiographs, due to the subtle soft tissue signs of fracture. Stress fractures, especially of the tibia head, may not demonstrate early osseous changes on x-ray and may require a bone scan for definitive diagnosis. Posterior dislocation of the shoulder and hand can be easily missed and should be suspected if a fall drives the humeral head backwards. If external rotation is impossible it's likely that posterior dislocation is to blame and surgical reduction may be necessary. Anterior cruciate ligament tears are easily overlooked, because as little as 5 mm of laxity is a positive finding on the Lachman test. Continued midfoot pain can

TABLE 13.4 Common Acute Sports Injuries

Injury	Symptom	Likely Resulting Problem
Blow to chest	Pop/pull with trunk rotation	Suspect strain
Blow to chest	Point tenderness	Suspect fracture or deep bruise
Blow or twisting to back	Severe pain, blood in urine	Suspect deep bruise, serious strain, kidney problem
New shoes	Posterior heel pain	Suspect retrocalcaneal bursitis
Blow to abdomen	Pain, guarding, shoulder pain	Suspect internal organ damage
Blow to abdomen	Mild pain, loss of breath, hyperventilation	Suspect contusion
Twisting of trunk	Soreness with movement	Suspect muscle strain
Sudden twisting of thigh	Pop or tearing with groin pain, worse with movement	Suspect groin strain
Finger/thumb compressed or twisted	Pain, able to make fist	Suspect contusion or sprain
Sudden run or jump	Pop/pull & pain posterior thigh	Suspect hamstring pull
Sudden run/jump/twist of knee	Pop/snap/locking/giving way, knee pain, deformity	Suspect internal tissue tear or damage

indicate a Lisfranc fracture instead of a severe sprain. Weight-bearing radiographs are best at demonstrating this fracture, which usually requires open reduction and internal fixation.

Common acute injuries are detailed in Table 13.4.

NURSING AND MEDICINE IGNORE MYTH AND PROMOTE MUSCULOSKELETAL HEALTH

It has been estimated that by the year 2030 the number of persons 65 years and older will reach 70 million in the U. S. (USDHHS, 1996a) which, if true, will produce approximately 42 million older adults engaging in various sports, fitness, or leisure time physical activi-

TABLE 13.5 Aerobic Exercise Training

	AHA	ACSM	CDC/ACSM	AACVPR
Frequency/wk	> or = 3	3 to 5	Daily	3 to 5
Intensity	50–60% max heart rate	55–90% max heart rate	Moderate	50% VO2max
Duration	30 minutes	15–16 minutes	30 minutes	30–45 minutes

AHA = American Heart Association, ACSM = American College of Sports Medicine, CDC = Centers for Disease Control, AACVPR = American Association for Cardiovascular and Pulmonary Rehabilitation

ties. Recognizing that advancing age and inactivity are associated with several chronic diseases, it is important to understand and utilize population-specific guidelines for aerobic, endurance, flexibility and resistance training. Modification of activity intensity and rapidity of progression (start low, go slow) are very important considerations when designing programs or counseling the aging athlete. From a safety standpoint, a greater variability in weights and resistance is necessary to accommodate the range of physiologic changes that occur during senescence.

Patients with significant medical history should be cleared by their personal physician for participation in either a formal supervised rehabilitation program or an independent program based on Tables 13.5 and 13.6 as tolerated. Research by Vander (1982) supports preparticipatory evaluation of previously sedentary older adults (men older than age 40 and women older than age 50) before beginning a vigorous physical activity program. He established a goal of more than 500 calories over basal requirements per week for patients older than 65. Longer warm-up and cool-down periods, with stretching, will prevent shortened, spastic muscles with workouts. Programs prescribed for competitive athletes are usually not appropriate for elderly persons.

The health history of an aging athlete is best taken with the traditional geriatric approach listed in here (Jaffe, 1992).

- Pace questions based on client ability and energy level.
- Make sure eyeglasses and hearing aid are worn.
- Use terms based on the age and education of the patient.

TABLE 13.6 Resistance Training

Specific Population	Repetitions	Number of exercises	Frequency
Healthy sedentary (Carpenter & Nelson, 1999)	1 set, 8–12 repetitions maximum	8–10 exercises	2–3 days/wk
Elderly or frail ACSM guideline	1 set, 10–15 repetitions	8–10 exercises	2–3 days/wk
Chronic low back pain (Carpenter & Nelson, 1999)	1 set, 8–15 repetitions maximum	Isolated lumbar extension exercises	1 day/wk
Cardiac patients AHA Class A & B (1999 AACVPR guideline)	1 set, 12–15 repetitions maximum	8–10 exercises	2–3 days/wk
Heart transplant recipients (Braith, 1998)	1 set, 10–15 repetitions maximum	8–10 exercises, isolated lumbar extension exercise	2 days/wk 1 day/wk

AHA = American Heart Association, ACSM = American College of Sports Medicine, CDC = Centers for Disease Control, AACVPR = American Association for Cardiovascular and Pulmonary Rehabilitation.

- Explain limitations caused by senescence.
- Use reminiscing and association techniques to elicit information.
- Use family members or friends to confirm pertinent history.
- Carefully document reports of chest pain, leg swelling, shortness of breath, exertional dyspnea, weight changes, reduced neurosensory perception, cognitive changes, skin wounds, foot changes, falls, trauma, impaired mobility, weakness, joint pain, and retirement/role changes.

Identifying previous exercise, sports, and leisure time physical activity will allow you to establish a baseline of intensity, frequency, and type of conditioning that the athlete has maintained. Often, the guidelines previously mentioned also help you to recommend incremental changes suitable for the senior's current health situation.

Alterations in balance, coordination, range of motion, fatigue, malaise, strength, pain, gait, rigidity, deformity, potential adverse drug reactions, polypharmacy and sleep patterns should be considered individually in the older sports participant(Loftis & Glover, 1993). Each of these items is addressed in convenient algorithmic form in Loftis and Glover's, *Decision Making in Gerontologic Nursing*.

SUMMARY AND CONCLUSION

Sports activities and regular exercise not only lengthen life but also enhance its quality by ameliorating many age-related declines in the musculoskeletal and cardiovascular systems. An awareness of the prevalence and importance of, and guidelines for exercise in older people should be reflected in our assessment, counseling and treatment. Everyone ages differently based on genetics, baseline fitness, and comorbidities. The exploding population of aging athletes necessitates a new look at senescence in America and a new approach to promoting fitness activities in the elderly. Seniors generally possess significant time to act on behalf of their health. Their commitment to exercise patterns can be easily reinforced because of the rapid benefits, such as enhanced functional independence, endurance, and self-esteem.

REFERENCES

Abdenour, T. E., & Thygerson, A. L. (1993). *Sports injury care.* New York: Mosby.

American College of Sports Medicine (1998). The recommended quality and quantity of exercise for developing and maintaining cardio respiratory and muscular fitness and flexibility in healthy adults. *Medical Science Sports & Exercise, 30,* 975–91.

Bellamy, N., Buchanan, W. W., & Goldsmith, C. H. (1988). Validation study of WOMAC: A health status instrument for measuring clinically important, patient relevant outcomes following total hip or knee arthroplasty in osteoarthritis. *Journal of Rheumatology, 1,* 95–108.Braith, R. W. (1998). Exercise training in patients with CHF and heart transplant recipients. *Medical Science Sports & Exercise, 30,* S367–S378.

Carpenter, D. & Nelson, B. (1999). Low back strengthening for health, rehabilitation, and injury prevention. *Medical Science Sports & Exercise, 31,* 18–24.

Cornoni-Huntley, J. C., Huntley, R. R., & Feldman, J. J. (1990). *Health status and well being of the elderly.* New York: Oxford University Press.

Cushnaghan, J., McCarthy, C., & Dieppe, P. (1994). Taping the patella medially—a new treatment for osteoarthritis of the knee joint. *British Medical Journal, 308,* 753–755.

Dambro, M. R. (1998). *Griffith's five minute clinical consult* (6th ed.). Baltimore, MD: Williams & Wilkins.

Dieppe, P., Chard, J., Failkner, A., & Lohmander, S. (2000). Musculoskeletal disorders. In S. Barton, C. Adams, L. G. Amore, G. Jones, N. Maskrey, & H. McConnell (Eds.), *Clinical evidence* (pp. 649–705). London: British Medical Journal Publishing Group.

Dishman, R. K. (1984). The determinants of physical activity and exercise. *Public Health Report, 100,* 158–171.

Fontane, P. E., & Hurd, P. D. (1992). Self perceptions of national senior olympians. *Behavior, Health and Aging, 2*(2), 101–110.

Feigenbaum, M. S., & Gentry, R. K. (2001). Prescription of resistance training for clinical populations. *The American Journal of Medicine & Sports, III*(III), 146–158.

Gaffney, K. L. (1995). Intra-articular triamcinalone hexacetonide in knee osteoarthritis: factors influencing the clinical response. *Annals of Rheumatic Disease, 54,* 379–81.

Hill, C. A. (2001, January/February). Caring for the aging athlete. *Geriatric Nursing, 22*(1), 43–45.

Hizon, J. W. (2001, May/June). Playing through the pain. *The American Journal of Medicine and Sports, III*(III), 186–187.

Jaffe, M. (1992). *Geriatric instant instructor.* Mexico City: Skidmore-Roth.

Kahn, R. L., & House, J. S. (1989). Age difference in productive activities. *Journal of Gerontology: Social Sciences, S129,* 44.

Kirkley, A., Websterbogaert, S., & Litchfield, R. (1999). The effect of bracing on varus gonarthrosis. *Journal of Bone Joint Surg, 81a,* 539–48.

Loftis, P. A., & Glover, T. L. (1993). *Decision making in gerontological nursing.* St. Louis: Mosby.

Meeusen, R. Van Der Veen, P. & Harley, S. (2001, May/Jun). Cold and compression in the treatment of athletic injuries. *The American Journal of Medicine & Sports, III*(III), 166–70.

Morris, M. (1997, February 21). U. S. senior sports classic VI comes to town. *Arizona Daily Star.*

Pavelka, J. K. (1995). Glycosaminoglycan polysulfuric acid in osteoarthritis of the knee. *Osteoarthritis Cartilage, 3,* 15–23.

Rodeheffer, R. J. (1984). Exercise cardiac output is maintained with advancing age in healthy human subjects: Cardiac dilatation and increased stroke volume compensate for diminished heart rate. *Circulation, 69,* 201–13.

Ross, P. D. (1996). Osteoporosis frequency, consequences and risk factors. *Archives of Internal Medicine, 156,* 1399–1411.

Rowe, J. W. (1990). Toward successful aging: limitation of the morbidity associated with normal aging. *Principles of Geriatric Medicine and Gerontology* (2nd ed.). New York: McGraw-Hill.

Schick, F. L., & Schick, R. (1994). *Statistical handbook on aging Americans.* Phoenix, AZ: Oryx.

Schumacher, H. R., Klippel, J. H., & Koopman, W. J. (1993). *Primer on the rheumatic diseases* (10th ed.). Atlanta, GA: Arthritis Foundation.

Scott, W. A. (1996). Injuries in active seniors. *The Physician and Sports Medicine, 24*(5), 2–8.

Scott, W. A., & Couzens, G. S. (1996). Treating injuries in active seniors. *Physical Sports Medicine, 24*(5).

U.S. Department of Health and Human Services (1991). *Health promotion and disease prevention* (supplement) *National health interview survey.* Rockville, MD: Author.

U.S. Department of Health and Human Services (1999). Physical activity and health: A report of the surgeon general. *U. S. Department of Health and Human Services, Centers for Disease Control and Prevention, National Center for Chronic Disease Prevention and Health Promotion,* 0–32. Rockville, MD: Author.

U.S. Department of Health and Human Services Public Health Service (2000). *Healthy people 2010.* Rockville, MD: Author.

Van Baar, M. E., Assendelft, W. J., & Dekker, J. (1999). Effectiveness of exercise therapy in patients with osteoarthritis of the hip or knee: a systematic review of randomized clinical trials. *Arthritis and Rheumatology, 42,* 1361–69.

Vander, L. (1982). Cardiovascular complications of recreational physical activity. *Physician Sports Medicine, 10,* 89–97.

Wallach, S. (1998). Osteoporosis. In M. R. Dambro (Ed.), *Griffith's 5 minute clinical consultant* (6th ed., pp. 752–53). Baltimore, MD: Williams & Wilkins.

Williams, R. A. (1999). *The athlete and heart disease.* Philadelphia: Lippincott, Williams & Wilkins.

Yelin, E., Henke, C., & Epstein, W. (1987). The work dynamics of the person with rheumatoid arthritis. *Arthritis and Rheumatology, 30,* 507–12.

Index

Springer Publishing Company

The Encyclopedia of Elder Care
The Comprehensive Resource on Geriatric and Social Care

Mathy D. Mezey, RN, EdD, FAAN, Editor-in-Chief
Barbara J. Berkman, DSW, **Christopher M. Callahan,** MD
Terry T. Fulmer, PhD, RN, FAAN, **Ethel L. Mitty,** EdD, RN
Gregory J. Paveza, MSW, PhD, **Eugenia L. Siegler,** MD, FACP,
Neville E. Strumpf, PhD, RN, FAAN, Associate Editors
Melissa M. Bottrell, MPH, PhDc, Managing Editor

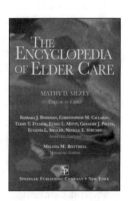

"**The Encyclopedia of Elder Care** *is an authoritative, comprehensive overview of the best clinical research and practice in contemporary gerontology and geriatrics. Editor Mathy D. Mezey, a distinguished pioneer in elder care, has been joined by many of the nation's most notable scholars and experienced clinicians in producing this timely, readable volume for an aging society.*"
—**George L. Maddox,** PhD

"**The Encyclopedia of Elder Care** *provides a valuable and far-ranging resource for professionals across the whole range of disciplines.*"
—**Bruce C. Vladeck,** PhD

Caring for elderly individuals requires a command of current information from multiple disciplines. Now, for the first time, this information has been gathered in a single source. Written by experts, this state-of-the-art resource features nearly 300 articles providing practical information on: home care; nursing home care; rehabilitation; case management; social services; assisted living; palliative care; and more. Each article concludes with references to pertinent Web Sites. Easy to read and extensively cross-referenced, the **Encyclopedia** is an indispensable tool for all in the caring professions.

2000   824pp   0-8261-1368-0   hardcover

536 Broadway, New York, NY 10012 • **Telephone: 212-431-4370**
Fax: 212-941-7842 • **Order Toll-Free: 877-687-7476**
Order On-line: www.springerpub.com

Springer Publishing Company

Emerging Infectious Diseases
Trends and Issues

Felissa R. Lashley, RN, PhD, ACRN, FAAN
Jerry D. Durham, RN, PhD, FAAN, Editors
Foreword by James M. Hughes, MD
Director of National Center for Infectious Diseases

Overuse of antibiotics, increased global air travel, and now terrorism, are
some of the reasons for the alarming increase in
new, antibiotic-resistant, or "conquered" infectious
diseases. This book provides health professionals,
especially nurses, with a broad overview of emerging and re-emerging diseases in the United States.
Written by a multidisciplinary group of nurses,
physicians, and infectious disease specialists, the
chapters detail   known outbreaks, symptoms,
sources of infection, modes of transmission, treatment, and prevention. The Appendix includes a
comprehensive resource list, including organizations and web sites.

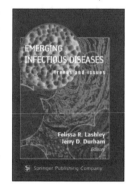

*"This book is a gem to read...It's an invaluable resource to clinicians and
educators who want a state-of-the-science reference for this fascinating and
important field."*
 —**Elaine Larson,** RN, PhD, FAAN, CIC, Columbia University

Partial Contents:

Background: Microbial Resistance to Antibiotics; Highlights of
 Significant Current EIDs.

Specific Diseases: Cholera; Cryptosporidiosis; Cyclospora cayetanensis;
 Dengue; Ebola, Marburg, and Lassa Fever; Escherichia coli O157:H7;
 Hantavirus; Hepatitis C; HIV/AIDS; Leginellosis; Lyme Disease;
 Malaria; Tuberculosis; Prion Diseases; Streptococcus pneumoniae;
 Enterococci; West Nile.

Special Considerations: Infection in Cancers and Chronic Diseases;
 Travel and EIDs; Immunocompromised Persons and EIDs;
 BioTerrorism; Behavioral and Cultural Aspects of Transmission.

2002   496pp 0-8261-1474-1   hard

536 Broadway, New York, NY 10012 • Telephone: 212-431-4370
Fax: 212-941-7842 • Order Toll-Free: 877-687-7476
Order On-line: www.springerpub.com